Essential Soaps

A Guide to Making Natural Soaps at Home

By
Well-Being Publishing

Copyright 2024 Well-Being Publishing. All rights reserved.

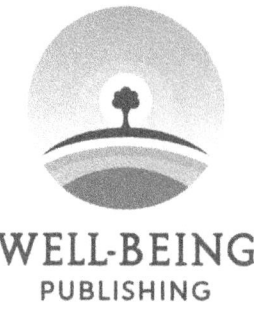

WELL-BEING
PUBLISHING

No part of this book may be reproduced in any form or by any electronic or mechanical means including information storage and retrieval systems, without permission in writing from the author. The only exception is by a reviewer, who may quote short excerpts in a review.

Although the author and publisher have made every effort to ensure that the information in this book was correct at press time, the author and publisher do not assume and hereby disclaim any liability to any party for any loss, damage, or disruption caused by errors or omissions, whether such errors or omissions result from negligence, accident, or any other cause.

This publication is designed to provide accurate and authoritative information with regard to the subject matter covered. It is sold with the understanding that the publisher is not engaged in rendering professional services. If legal advice or other expert assistance is required, the services of a competent professional should be sought.

The fact that an organization or website is referred to in this work as a citation and/or a potential source of further information does not mean that the author or the publisher endorses the information the organization or website may provide or recommendations it may make.

Please remember that Internet websites listed in this work may have changed or disappeared between when this work was written and when it is read.

To you,

Thank you!

Table of Contents

Introduction 1

Chapter 1: The Art of Soapmaking 5
    Understanding the Soapmaking Process 5
    The History of Soap: From Ancient to Modern Times 8

Chapter 2: Preparing Your Soapmaking Space 12
    Gathering Essential Equipment 12
    Safety Measures and Best Practices 15

Chapter 3: Basic Ingredients for Natural Soapmaking 19
    Oils, Butters, and Fats 19
    Lye Safety and Handling 23
    The Role of Water in Soapmaking 25

Chapter 4: Designing Your Soap Recipes 29
    Calculating Lye and Oil Ratios 29
    Customizing Soap Properties 33
    Recipe Formulation Tips and Tricks 36

Chapter 5: The Melt and Pour Method 40
    Getting Started with Melt and Pour 40
    Creative Designs and Techniques 43
    Adding Herbs, Colorants, and Textures 47

Chapter 6: Cold Process Soapmaking 51
    Step-by-Step Guide to Cold Process 51
    Creating Texture and Layers 53
    Swirling and Patterning Techniques 56

Chapter 7: Hot Process Soapmaking 61
    The Basics of Hot Process 61
    Crock Pot and Oven Methods 64
    Finishing Touches for Hot Process Soaps 67

Chapter 8: Superfatting and Saponification Explained 71
    Saponification Values and Why They Matter 71
    Benefits of Superfatting Your Soap 75

Chapter 9: Essential Oils and Aromatherapy in Soapmaking 78
    Essential Oil Safety and Usage 78
    Blending Essential Oils for Fragrance 81

Chapter 10: Herbal Additives and Botanicals 84
    Infusing Oils With Herbs 84
    Selecting and Using Dried Herbs and Flowers 88

Chapter 11: Natural Colorants and Clays 92
    Using Clays for Color and Texture 92
    Plant-Based Colorants: Roots, Berries, and Leaves 95

Chapter 12: Exfoliants and Texturizers 99
    Choosing the Right Exfoliant 99
    Incorporating Seeds, Salts, and Powders 102

Chapter 13: Milk Soaps and Alternative Liquids 106
    Making Soap with Milk 106
    Using Teas, Juices, and Other Liquids 109

Chapter 14: Vegan and Palm-Free Soap Options 113
    Plant-Based Soap Recipes 113
    Sustainable Alternatives to Palm Oil 116

Chapter 15: Speciality Soaps and Techniques 120
    Shampoo Bars and Conditioner Soaps 120
    Shaving Soaps and Scrub Bars 123

Chapter 16: Soap for Babies and Sensitive Skin 128

    Gentle Formulas and Hypoallergenic Ingredients 128
    Unscented and Soothing Soaps 132

Chapter 17: Themed and Seasonal Soapmaking 137
    Holiday and Celebration Soaps 137
    Creating a Seasonal Soap Line 141

Chapter 18: Packaging and Presentation 145
    Eco-Friendly Packaging Options 145
    Labeling Regulations and Best Practices 148

Chapter 19: Troubleshooting Common Soapmaking Issues 153
    Dealing with Acceleration and Ricing 153
    Preventing and Fixing Soda Ash 156

Chapter 20: Advanced Soapmaking Designs 159
    Embedding and Layering Techniques 159
    Mastering the In-The-Pot Swirl 163

Chapter 21: Scaling Up: Tips for Larger Batches 167
    Equipment for Bigger Batches 167
    Consistency and Quality Control 171

Chapter 22: Selling Your Handmade Soaps 175
    Setting Up a Soapmaking Business 175
    Marketing and Selling Online 179

Chapter 23: The Future of Soapmaking 182
    Trends in Natural Soapmaking 182
    Innovation and Sustainability in the Industry 185

Chapter 24: Joining the Soapmaking Community 190
    Forums, Workshops, and Events 190
    Collaborations and Networking 194

Chapter 25: Continuing Your Soapmaking Journey 197
    Further Education and Resources 197
    Experimentation and Ongoing Learning 200

    Online Review Request for This Book 203
Conclusion 204
Appendix A: Resource Directory 207
    Soapmaking Supplies and Ingredients 207
    Essential Oils and Natural Additives 207
    Packaging and Presentation 208
    Soapmaking Communities and Forums 208
    Workshops and Certifications 209
    Books and Publications 209
    Online Learning and Tutorials 209
Glossary of Soapmaking Terms 210

Introduction

Welcome to a world brimming with aromatic possibilities and creative adventure: natural soapmaking with herbs and essential oils. If you've ever marveled at the silkiness of a handmade soap or breathed deeply the calming blend of lavender and chamomile, you're in the right place. This book is your guide to crafting soap that delights the senses while promoting sustainable and eco-friendly practices. Whether you're a passionate DIY enthusiast, an aspiring small business owner, or someone simply intrigued by the art of soapmaking, this journey is for you.

Soapmaking isn't just a craft; it's an alchemy where science meets artistry, and the mundane transforms into the magnificent. By combining the right ingredients, temperatures, and techniques, you can create something truly magical. As we delve into this incredible world, you'll discover how natural ingredients can nourish not only your skin but also your soul. We'll guide you on how to blend essential oils for therapeutic benefits, infuse oils with vibrant herbs, and experiment with a myriad of textures and colors.

More than ever, people are seeking ways to reduce their environmental footprint and make healthier lifestyle choices. This shift towards sustainability and wellness makes handcrafted soap a perfect outlet for those values. In making your own soap, you gain complete control over the ingredients, allowing you to eliminate harmful chemicals and artificial additives while embracing the goodness of nature.

Well-Being Publishing

This book is structured to cater to all levels of soapmaking expertise. If you're just getting started, Chapter 1 will walk you through the basics, providing you with a solid foundation in understanding the soapmaking process. We'll explore the history of soap, tracing its evolution from ancient times to the present, illustrating how this humble product has remained a staple in human hygiene for millennia.

Adequate preparation is key to successful soapmaking. Setting up your workspace correctly, as outlined in Chapter 2, ensures a safe and efficient environment. Gathering the right equipment and understanding best practices minimizes mishaps and sets the stage for a smooth soapmaking experience.

Chapter 3 delves into the essential ingredients required to create natural soap. Oils, butters, and fats form the backbone of your soap, while lye acts as the catalyst that transforms these ingredients into the luxurious bars you'll soon be crafting. Understanding the role of water and learning how to handle lye safely are crucial skills you'll master.

Designing your soap recipes, discussed in Chapter 4, opens up a realm of creativity. It's where science and art intermingle; you'll learn to calculate lye and oil ratios and customize your soap's properties to meet your specific needs. This chapter is brimming with tips and tricks to help you formulate recipes that balance functionality with beauty.

For those keen on diving straight into the creative side, Chapters 5 through 7 cover various soapmaking methods. From the simplicity and immediacy of the Melt and Pour method to the nuanced techniques of Cold Process soapmaking and the rustic appeal of Hot Process soap, you're bound to find a method that resonates with your style and preferences.

Understanding the science behind soapmaking enhances your ability to innovate and troubleshoot effectively. Chapter 8 explains saponification and superfatting, integral elements that impact the final quality of your soap. These foundational concepts are elucidated in clear, practical terms to ensure even the novice soapmaker feels confident.

Fragrance plays a crucial role in the sensory appeal of your soap. In Chapter 9, you'll delve into the world of essential oils and their aromatic properties. Learn how to blend oils for unique scents and understand the safety guidelines to follow. Aromatherapy enthusiasts will find this chapter particularly enriching, unlocking the ability to craft soaps that do more than just cleanse—they heal and uplift.

Chapter 10 expands on the use of herbs and botanicals, offering techniques for infusing oils and utilizing dried herbs and flowers in your soaps. The use of natural colorants and clays, detailed in Chapter 11, allows you to add a visual appeal and textural diversity that elevate your creations from ordinary to extraordinary.

Sustainability is a recurring theme throughout this book. In Chapter 14, we address vegan and palm-free soap options, emphasizing eco-conscious choices that align with modern ethical considerations. You'll find plant-based recipes and sustainable alternatives that ensure your soapmaking process is both kind to the earth and compassionate to all living beings.

Of course, soapmaking extends beyond personal use. If you're considering turning your passion into a business, Chapter 22 provides insights into setting up a soapmaking enterprise, marketing, and selling online. It's packed with practical advice to help you navigate the entrepreneurial landscape, from initial planning to establishing a loyal customer base.

In the final chapters, you'll explore advanced techniques, troubleshoot common issues, and learn about packaging and presentation. These sections offer valuable knowledge even to experienced soapmakers, ensuring your skills and products continue to evolve.

As you embark on this journey, remember that soapmaking is not just about the end product; it's an enriching process that fosters creativity, mindfulness, and sustainability. We're excited to guide you through the art and science of soapmaking, helping you craft not just bars of soap, but pieces of art that embody your values and vision. Let's start this journey of discovery, one lather at a time.

Chapter 1:
The Art of Soapmaking

Soapmaking is more than a mere craft; it's an alchemical blend of science and artistry that transforms everyday ingredients into luxurious bars of pure goodness. From the delicate blend of oils and lye to the meticulous layering of fragrances and botanicals, each step in the process invites both creativity and precision. This chapter will introduce you to the enchanting world of handcrafted soaps, tracing the evolution and significance of soap through history while demystifying the process that turns raw materials into skin-loving cleansers. Whether you're an eager beginner or a seasoned artisan, our aim is to inspire and equip you with the knowledge to create soaps that are not only beautiful and aromatic but also sustainable and kind to the Earth. As you embark on this soapy journey, you'll discover that soapmaking is an art form that nurtures both the mind and soul, offering endless possibilities for innovation and personal expression.

Understanding the Soapmaking Process

The Soapmaking Process is essential for anyone who wants to immerse themselves in the art and science of crafting natural soaps. At its core, soapmaking is a fascinating blend of chemistry and creativity. The basic principle involves combining oils and fats (often called lipids) with an alkaline substance (commonly known as lye) to produce a chemical reaction called saponification. While this sounds scientific, it's something crafters have been doing for centuries with often rudimentary tools. By understanding this process, you'll be able to create soaps that not only cleanse but also nourish and delight the senses.

The first step in soapmaking involves choosing your oils, butters, and fats. These ingredients form the backbone of your soap and affect its texture, hardness, lather, and moisturizing properties. Oils like olive, coconut, and palm are common choices, but the possibilities are almost endless. Each oil has a unique combination of fatty acids, and these contribute different qualities to the final product. For instance, coconut oil is excellent for producing a rich, bubbly lather, while olive oil yields a gentle, moisturizing bar. The beauty of soapmaking lies in tailoring these ingredients to suit your personal preferences or specific skin needs.

The next critical component is lye, which is either sodium hydroxide (for solid soap) or potassium hydroxide (for liquid soap). When lye is mixed with water and combined with fats, the saponification process begins, transforming these ingredients into soap. Handling lye requires careful attention to safety, as it is a caustic substance. Proper protective gear, such as gloves and goggles, is essential. Despite its intimidating nature, lye is indispensable to soapmaking, and with respectful handling, it becomes just another part of your creative toolkit.

Saponification is the true heart of the soapmaking process. As the lye solution interacts with the fats, a series of chemical reactions occur, breaking down the triglycerides in the oils and forming soap and glycerin. This transformation can take from a few hours to several days, depending on the method used. During saponification, the soap mixture goes through distinct phases—first becoming a thick, custard-like "trace," and then hardening into a solid bar. Monitoring and understanding these stages are crucial as they affect the final qualities of your soap.

Essential Soaps

The choice of method also plays a significant role in the soapmaking process. The three primary methods are cold process, hot process, and melt and pour. Each has its benefits and drawbacks. The cold process method involves mixing oils and lye at room temperature and pouring the mixture into molds to cure for four to six weeks. This method allows for intricate designs and the use of delicate essential oils and botanicals but requires patience. In contrast, the hot process method accelerates saponification by applying heat, either in a crock pot or oven, reducing curing time but making the soap more rustic in appearance. Meanwhile, the melt and pour method involves pre-made soap bases that can be melted, colored, and fragranced before being remolded, making it ideal for beginners or those short on time.

Once saponification is complete, the curing process begins, especially crucial for cold process soaps. Curing allows the soap to harden and the excess moisture to evaporate, which improves the bar's longevity and performance. This step takes place in a cool, dry environment and can last several weeks. During curing, the soap's pH levels stabilize, resulting in a milder, more skin-friendly bar.

It's also important to consider the creative aspects of soapmaking. Adding herbs, essential oils, and natural colorants can elevate your soap from merely functional to a work of art. Herbs can infuse your soap with beneficial properties, such as soothing lavender or invigorating peppermint. Essential oils provide natural fragrance and bring aromatherapy benefits. Natural colorants, like clays, root powders, and plant extracts, can transform the appearance of your soap, creating visually stunning bars that are also kind to the skin. The right combination of these additives can turn a standard bar of soap into a unique and luxurious product that reflects your personal style and ethos.

Understanding the science and nuances of the soapmaking process empowers you to experiment and develop your unique recipes. This knowledge serves as the foundation for exploring more complex techniques, such as layering, swirling, and texturing, covered in later chapters. As you gain confidence, you can push the boundaries of traditional soapmaking, creating bars that are not only effective but also beautiful and unique.

In conclusion, mastering the soapmaking process is an exciting journey of discovery. It's a harmonious blend of precision and creativity, where science meets art. With a solid grasp of this fundamental process, you're well on your way to crafting beautiful, natural soaps that reflect your style and values. Embrace the learning curve, enjoy the process, and let your imagination soar. With practice and persistence, you'll soon be creating soaps that are both a joy to use and to share.

The History of Soap: From Ancient to Modern Times

This history provides a fascinating glimpse into the evolution of a product that's become a staple in our lives. Soap, in its simplest form, is a combination of an acid and a base resulting in a salt. This process, known as saponification, appears to have roots as far back as 2800 BCE in ancient Babylon. Here, archeologists discovered a clay cylinder inscribed with a formula for soap made from fats boiled with ashes. Such early records suggest that soap in its rudimentary form was primarily used for cleaning wool and cotton in preparation for weaving rather than for personal hygiene.

Moving forward in history, we find soap becoming more refined and gaining a foothold in early civilizations. The ancient Egyptians, renowned for their advances in medicine and lifestyle sophistication, documented the use of a soap-like substance to prepare wool for weaving and as a treatment for skin diseases. Their concoctions often included a mix of animal and vegetable oils with alkaline salts, indicating a significant understanding of saponification. Ancient papyri and hieroglyphs provide evidence that soap was also used in personal cleanliness, albeit more as a luxury item for the elite.

The Romans further innovated soapmaking, adopting the usage of soap for personal hygiene and therapeutic purposes. Pliny the Elder, in his "Natural History," recorded that both the Gauls and Germans used a soap made from tallow and ashes. Excavations in Pompeii have uncovered an entire soap factory, suggesting a thriving industry. The Roman approach to cleanliness, emphasizing daily baths in sophisticated bathhouses, highlighted the importance of soap in their culture. However, after the fall of Rome, Europe saw a decline in soap use, linked to the broader regression in sanitary practices during the Dark Ages.

Interestingly, the Islamic Golden Age was a period of advancement in soapmaking. Innovators in the Middle East experimented with different ingredients, such as olive oil and alkaline substances derived from plants. From cities like Nablus, Kufa, and Basra, soap production techniques spread throughout the Islamic world and into medieval Europe later. Various soaps, known for their distinctive scents and cleansing properties, emerged, with Castile soap from Spain being one of the most famous. This era focused on the use of high-quality, pure ingredients, setting a standard that would influence soapmaking practices for centuries to come.

As Europe emerged from the Middle Ages, soapmaking began to flourish again. Guilds formed in cities like Marseilles, producing soap using new and improved methods. French soapmakers in the 16th century perfected the process, using olive oil instead of animal fats, along with seaweed-derived soda ash. The Marseilles soap became famed for its quality and purity. Around the same time, in England, soap became more accessible to the public, though heavy taxation in the 17th century made it a luxury for many until duties were lifted in the 19th century.

The Industrial Revolution marked a monumental shift in soapmaking. With the development of large-scale manufacturing processes and the chemical industry, soap became more affordable and widely available. One significant milestone was Michel Eugène Chevreul's discovery in 1823 of the chemical nature of fats, which laid the groundwork for the modern soapmaking process. Parallelly, in 1791, the Frenchman Nicolas Leblanc developed a method to produce sodium carbonate (soda ash) from common salt, providing a key ingredient for soap production. These advancements moved soap from artisanal craftsmanship into mass production.

In the United States, soap manufacturers like Procter & Gamble rose to prominence in the 19th century, capitalizing on these technological advancements. They utilized by-products from the slaughterhouses to produce soap on an industrial scale. Iconic soaps like Ivory, which was marketed as a pure and floating soap, highlighted innovation in both product development and marketing strategies. These companies transformed soap from a luxury into an everyday household necessity, revolutionizing the way society approached cleanliness and hygiene.

During the 20th and 21st centuries, soapmaking has seen a renaissance of sorts, particularly among DIY enthusiasts and small-scale artisans. As awareness of environmental issues and the impact of synthetic chemicals on health has grown, so has the demand for natural, handmade soaps. Modern soapmakers echo the ancient techniques, using traditional fats and oils, but with a new emphasis on sustainability and eco-friendly practices. From organic oils to essential oils and botanicals, today's soap is as much about artistry and sustainable living as it is about cleanliness.

In conclusion, the journey of soap from ancient Babylonian clay tablets to today's artisanal bars is a testament to human ingenuity and the quest for improved health and hygiene. Understanding this rich history not only deepens our appreciation for the humble bar of soap but also inspires us to carry forward the tradition of craftsmanship, sustainability, and innovation in soapmaking. Whether you are a hobbyist or an aspiring soap entrepreneur, this historical knowledge provides a solid foundation upon which you can build your own soapmaking legacy.

Chapter 2: Preparing Your Soapmaking Space

Creating the perfect soapmaking space is more than just setting up a workstation; it's about fostering an environment where creativity and precision can flourish. First, designate a well-ventilated area that has ample counter space to lay out all your materials and equipment. Make sure your workspace is free from distractions and easy to clean, as soapmaking can get messy. Organize your essential tools—molds, mixing bowls, thermometers, and scales—so they are easily accessible. Safety should be your top priority; have safety goggles, gloves, and long sleeves on hand to protect against potential lye splashes. If you're working with essential oils, ventilation is crucial to disperse any strong scents. Lastly, having a dedicated soapmaking area not only streamlines the process but also sets the stage for your soapmaking journey to be a fulfilling and enjoyable experience. Each batch you create will reflect the care and thoughtfulness you put into preparing your workspace.

Gathering Essential Equipment

This is the cornerstone of creating your own soapmaking workspace. Having the right tools and equipment not only enhances your soapmaking experience but also ensures safety and efficiency. From basic tools to specialized gadgets, this section is your comprehensive guide to gathering everything you need to get started.

First off, let's talk about the basics that you simply can't do without. A digital scale is an absolute must-have; precision is paramount in soapmaking. Even slight deviations in measurements can significantly alter the final product. Opt for a scale that measures in both grams and ounces for versatility. You're going to be measuring oils, butters, lye, and other ingredients, so a good, reliable scale is non-negotiable.

Another essential item is a well-made, heat-resistant container for handling lye. Stainless steel or heavy-duty plastic are your best bets here. Make sure the container is large enough to hold your lye solution without sloshing and stable enough to avoid tipping over. Trust me, a good, stable container can prevent a lot of potential accidents.

Measuring cups and spoons come next. These aren't your kitchen ones; you'll want to invest in a dedicated set for soapmaking. Materials like stainless steel or polypropylene are excellent choices because they're resistant to lye corrosion. Easily distinguishable and preferably color-coded measuring cups and spoons can speed up your process and reduce errors.

Mixing vessels and stirring tools are also high on the list. You'll need large, heat-resistant bowls for mixing your oils and lye solution. Stainless steel bowls are generally preferred, as they won't react with your ingredients. For stirring, silicone spatulas and stainless steel whisks are both excellent choices. They're easy to clean and durable, standing up to the rigorous demands of soapmaking.

Once you're ready to blend, an immersion blender, also known as a stick blender, becomes indispensable. This tool dramatically cuts down the time required to bring your soap mixture to trace—a crucial state where the soap thickens to the point of leaving a trace when drizzled on its surface. A good immersion blender can save you a lot of time and elbow grease, making the process significantly smoother.

Molds are, of course, essential for shaping your soap. Silicone molds are incredibly popular among soapmakers because they make unmolding a breeze and come in a range of shapes and sizes. Wooden molds are another great option, especially for larger batches, but remember to line them with freezer paper to prevent sticking. It's also handy to have a supply of small molds for sample-sized soaps or test batches.

Of course, safety gear cannot be overlooked. Lye is a hazardous material, and proper safety equipment is critical. At the very least, you'll need safety goggles, long sleeves, and rubber gloves to protect your skin and eyes from splashes and spills. A well-ventilated area or a fume hood can mitigate the risk from fumes during lye solution preparation. Don't skimp on safety—it's an integral part of your soapmaking kit.

If you plan to experiment with different colors, textures, and fragrances, additional gear will be necessary. Pipettes for precise measurements of essential oils, small bowls or ramekins for mixing colors, and dedicated small whisks or spoons are invaluable in this area. Having these tools ready will make your creative process smoother and more enjoyable.

Thermometers are another critical tool, especially if you're working with cold process or hot process methods where temperature control can affect saponification. An instant-read digital thermometer provides quick and accurate readings, helping you to ensure that your lye and oils are at the right temperature before mixing.

If you're serious about soapmaking as a business or a passionate hobby, a soap cutter is a great investment. Whether you choose a simple wire cutter or a more complex multi-wire model, a dedicated soap cutter helps you achieve clean, uniform bars of soap every time. Consistency is key, especially if you're planning to sell your soaps.

Last but certainly not least, cleaning supplies. Dedicated sponges, scrubbing brushes, and cleaning cloths that you use exclusively for your soap equipment will make the post-soapmaking cleanup easier and safer. Remember to never use these tools for food preparation afterward.

Gathering your essential equipment might seem like a daunting task, but having the right tools at your disposal can transform your soapmaking journey from a challenging endeavor to a joyful and creative experience. As you become more familiar with the soapmaking process, you may find yourself adding more niche tools and gadgets to suit your particular style and preferences. The investment in high-quality equipment pays dividends in the quality of your final product and the efficiency of your process.

Embarking on your soapmaking adventure armed with the right equipment sets a solid foundation for success. This journey is as much about enjoying the process as it is about the final product. Well-equipped, you're now ready to dive into the fascinating world of crafting your own unique, natural soaps. Let your creativity flow, and your soapmaking experience will be both safe and immensely rewarding.

Safety Measures and Best Practices

Safety is absolutely paramount in soapmaking. Whether you're a seasoned soapmaker or a beginner, ensuring safety in your workspace and in handling materials can make or break your experience. Without proper precautions, the beautiful art of soapmaking can quickly turn into a hazardous activity. So, let's delve into the critical aspects you must consider to maintain a safe and efficient soapmaking environment.

To start off, always make sure that your soapmaking area is well-ventilated. Lye, a key ingredient in the saponification process, can emit fumes that are not safe to inhale in a confined space. Open windows and use fans to facilitate proper airflow. It's not just about avoiding discomfort; it's about preventing potential respiratory issues.

Another foundational element of soapmaking safety is the use of personal protective equipment (PPE). This includes gloves, goggles, and long sleeves. Lye is caustic, and any direct contact can lead to chemical burns. Safety goggles protect your eyes from accidental splashes, while gloves and long sleeves guard your skin.

It's also advisable to keep a spray bottle of vinegar nearby. If any lye solution spills on your skin, vinegar can neutralize the alkali. But remember, this is just a first-aid measure. Immediate flushing with plenty of water is crucial to mitigate the effects of contact.

Proper storage of materials also plays a significant role in safety. Lye should be stored in a high, dry place, away from children, pets, and any moisture. The same goes for essential oils and other additives, many of which can be harmful if ingested or improperly handled. Clear labeling of all substances will help prevent any dangerous mix-ups.

When weighing and measuring ingredients, accuracy is crucial—not just for the quality of your soap but for your safety as well. Using accurate digital scales ensures that you're working with the correct amounts, particularly when handling lye. Too much or too little can lead to soap that's either too harsh or fails to saponify properly.

Let's talk about the mixing process. Always add lye to water, never the reverse. Adding water to lye can cause a violent reaction, leading to splatters and possible burns. Also, use heat-resistant containers for mixing lye since the mixture will become very hot. Glass, plastic, or certain types of silicone are safest.

Regarding workspace cleanliness, this cannot be overstated. Keeping your workspace clean and organized prevents accidents and contamination. Clean spills immediately, and use dedicated tools and equipment for soapmaking to avoid cross-contamination with food or other substances. An untidy workspace is a breeding ground for mistakes.

It's also a good practice to understand and follow all safety guidelines specific to the ingredients you're using. Essential oils, for example, vary greatly in terms of their safe usage rates. Some can cause skin irritation if used in high concentrations, while others might have restrictions based on age or health conditions. Knowing these details can prevent allergic reactions or other health issues.

Disposal of waste materials is another aspect often overlooked. Ensure that leftover lye or lye-water mixtures are properly diluted and neutralized before disposing of them. Improper disposal can harm the environment and pose risks to others.

If you're working on a soapmaking project that involves children or pets around, it's crucial to set up barriers to keep them out of the soapmaking area. Curious hands or paws can lead to serious accidents. Educate older children about the dangers and make sure they understand the importance of not touching your materials or equipment.

Consider keeping a first aid kit nearby, stocked with essentials like bandages, antiseptic solutions, and burn creams. While everyone hopes never to use it, having it on hand means you're prepared for any minor mishaps that might occur.

Once your soapmaking session is complete, the safety measures don't end there. Labeling is crucial, especially if you're setting soaps aside to cure. Clearly marked soap batches help you keep track of curing times and ingredients used, which is especially important if you're producing multiple formulations at once.

Let's not forget about ongoing education. The soapmaking community is vast and knowledgeable, and staying updated on best practices and potential hazards is key to maintaining safety. Forums, workshops, and courses can provide new safety insights and reinforce what you already know.

Lastly, maintain a mindset of continuous improvement. Regularly assess your setup and practices to identify potential hazards or inefficiencies. Even small changes can make a big difference in creating a safer, more enjoyable soapmaking experience.

In conclusion, integrating thorough safety measures and best practices in your soapmaking process isn't just about following rules—it's about creating an environment where creativity and passion can flourish without risk. As you continue your journey in soapmaking, let safety be your constant companion, ensuring that every bar crafted is not only a piece of art but also a testament to your commitment to responsible crafting.

Chapter 3: Basic Ingredients for Natural Soapmaking

Mastering the art of natural soapmaking starts with understanding your basic ingredients. The building blocks of any great soap are a carefully chosen blend of oils, butters, and fats, which contribute to the soap's texture, lather, and moisturizing properties. Equally important is lye, a critical component in the chemical reaction known as saponification that transforms fats and oils into soap. Handling lye requires strict safety measures, as it is a highly caustic substance, but rest assured, with proper precautions, it can be managed effectively. Water is another fundamental ingredient, acting as the medium that dissolves the lye and facilitates the saponification process. Each of these ingredients brings its own unique properties to the table, forming the foundation upon which your natural, eco-friendly soap creations are built.

Oils, Butters, and Fats

These form the cornerstone of natural soapmaking. These ingredients are the backbone of your soap's structure, texture, and skin-loving properties. When chosen thoughtfully, they can elevate a simple bar of soap into a luxurious, nourishing experience. Whether you're a seasoned soapmaker or just starting out, understanding the variety and benefits of different oils, butters, and fats is crucial.

First, let's talk about *carrier oils*. These oils are liquid at room temperature and form the bulk of your soap's base. Common carrier oils include olive oil, coconut oil, and canola oil. Olive oil is a favorite for its moisturizing properties and creamy lather. Conversely, coconut oil provides excellent cleansing power and boosts the soap's lather dramatically, though it can be drying, so it's often balanced with other oils.

Naturally, there's more to oils than just olive and coconut. *Sweet almond oil* and *jojoba oil* are fantastic additions for their skin-conditioning properties. If you've ever felt the luxuriousness of an almond oil massage, you know what an amazing ingredient this can be. Jojoba oil, which closely resembles the natural sebum of your skin, is exceptionally moisturizing and non-greasy.

Next up are the lush *butters*. Shea butter and cocoa butter are perhaps the most commonly used. Shea butter lends a creamy, stable lather and adds to your soap's hardness. It's rich in vitamins and fatty acids, making it nourishing for your skin. Cocoa butter, on the other hand, provides emollient properties, giving your soap a velvety smooth texture. It's particularly beneficial for dry skin, given its rich, moisturizing qualities.

Then, we have mango butter, which offers a blend of stability and emulsification. It's less greasy compared to shea or cocoa butter, making it a great choice for those who prefer a lighter feel on the skin. Mango butter can also contribute to a harder bar of soap, which is always a plus when you want your creations to last longer.

In addition to soft oils and butters, you might also consider using *hard fats*. *Palm oil* is traditional in many soap recipes due to its ability to create firm bars that lather well. However, given environmental concerns, many soapmakers are turning to sustainable palm oil or alternatives like tallow and lard. Tallow, rendered from beef fat, and lard, rendered from pork fat, are classical soapmaking ingredients that produce exceptionally creamy lather and hard, long-lasting bars of soap.

If animal products are not your thing, consider using *castor oil* as a vegan alternative. Castor oil is a superstar in soapmaking, known for boosting lather and adding moisture. Just a small amount can significantly enhance the benefits of your soap. It's thick and sticky, meaning it helps hold the soap together, resulting in bars that don't melt away quickly.

Balancing these oils, butters, and fats is an art form in itself. Each brings unique properties that contribute to the overall character of the soap. Some oils are better for lather, like coconut and castor oil. Some are quintessential for hardness, like palm oil or tallow. Others, such as olive and jojoba oil, are ideal for moisturizing.

Understanding *fatty acid profiles* will help you make informed decisions when designing your soap recipes. For example, oleic acid, found abundantly in olive oil, provides conditioning properties. Lauric acid, predominant in coconut oil, is great for lather and cleansing. Stearic acid, found in butters like shea and cocoa, contributes to a hard, stable bar, while linoleic acid, found in oils like sunflower and hemp, offers skin-conditioning benefits.

Temperature control is another factor to consider when using various fats and butters. Ingredients like shea butter and cocoa butter have higher melting points, which means that special attention is needed during the soapmaking process to ensure they blend seamlessly with your other oils. It's often best to melt these butters gently and incorporate them into your oil mixture to prevent any grittiness in the final soap.

Moreover, sourcing quality ingredients is crucial. Opt for organic and unrefined oils and butters wherever possible. These not only contribute to a purer final product but also retain more of their inherent benefits. For instance, unrefined shea butter still contains high levels of vitamins and nutrients that refined versions may lack.

Crafting your own unique soap blend involves a bit of trial and error. Don't be afraid to experiment with different ratios and combinations of oils, butters, and fats. Each batch of soap you make is an opportunity to learn and refine your recipes. Keep detailed notes of your ingredients and their proportions, so you can replicate successful batches and adjust those that didn't turn out quite as planned.

It's also essential to consider the ecological impact of your ingredient choices. Sustainable practices are more than just a trend; they are a responsibility for all of us soil-makers. Palm oil is a versatile and valuable soapmaking ingredient, but always look for suppliers who provide sustainably harvested options. Moving towards more sustainable fats like coconut oil, olive oil, and even innovative options like algae-based oils can make a significant difference.

Finally, as you gain confidence and skill, think about the additional benefits these oils, butters, and fats can provide beyond their basic properties. Shea butter is not just moisturizing but also soothing and anti-inflammatory, making it great for sensitive skin. Olive oil is packed with antioxidants like vitamin E, which help to maintain the skin's barrier and calm irritation. These added benefits can become the selling points of your soaps, making them not just cleansing bars but therapeutic luxuries.

Remember, the journey of formulating your perfect soap is as rewarding as the destination. Embrace the process of discovery, let your creativity flow, and take pride in the natural, eco-friendly products you create. Each bar of soap crafted with care and intention is not only a testament to your skills but also to your commitment to sustainability and well-being.

Lye Safety and Handling

The safe handling of lye is absolutely crucial when you're delving into the world of soapmaking. Lye, chemically known as sodium hydroxide when solidified or potassium hydroxide when in liquid form, is a potent substance that demands respect and careful handling. This section's intent is to provide you with the knowledge required to handle lye safely, allowing you to enjoy the wonderful process of crafting natural soaps without unnecessary risks.

Lye is essential in soapmaking because it initiates the chemical reaction known as saponification, which transforms oils and fats into soap. Despite its importance, lye is highly caustic and can cause severe burns upon contact with skin or eyes. It can also produce harmful fumes when it reacts with water. This is why a dedicated, well-ventilated workspace and proper protective gear are non-negotiable when working with lye.

Before you even think of opening that container of lye, make sure you've got the right safety gear. Wear long sleeves, gloves, safety goggles, and a mask or respirator to protect yourself from splashes and fumes. Working in a well-ventilated area or near an open window can reduce the risk of inhaling lye dust or fumes. Setting up a dedicated, clutter-free lye mixing space will help avoid spills and keep accidents to a minimum.

Always add lye to water and never the other way around. Adding water to lye can cause a volatile reaction, sometimes leading to an explosive situation. The correct method is to slowly sprinkle lye into the water while stirring gently. You'll notice the mixture heating up and emitting fumes, so it's important to do this step in a well-ventilated area. It's wise to use a dedicated heat-resistant container for this purpose; stainless steel or heavy-duty plastic works best.

One of the most nerve-wracking moments for beginners is the initial lye mixing. This should ideally be done outdoors or under a fume hood. When mixing, make sure not to lean directly over the container to avoid inhaling the fumes. Stir slowly and gently until the lye is completely dissolved. You'll feel the container heat up almost instantly due to the exothermic reaction between the lye and water. Let the lye solution cool down to the desired temperature before mixing it with oils.

Storage of lye is the next critical element in maintaining a safe working environment. Always store lye in its original container, tightly sealed, and out of reach of children and pets. Consider labeling the container clearly with warnings and storing it in a locked cabinet. Make sure the area where you store the lye is cool and dry to avoid any unwanted reactions. Humidity can cause lye to clump together or form a crust, which can be problematic during measurement.

Accidents can happen, despite our best precautions. Knowing how to respond quickly can make all the difference. If lye comes into contact with your skin or eyes, rinse immediately with copious amounts of water and seek medical attention if necessary. Keep a bottle of vinegar handy; although it won't neutralize lye on skin, it can help neutralize small spills on surfaces. Always have your phone nearby to call for help in case of a serious incident, and never work with lye when you're alone at home.

Cleaning up after a lye mixing session should be approached with the same level of caution. Use separate utensils and containers exclusively for soapmaking to avoid cross-contamination. After you're done with the lye solution, wash everything thoroughly with plenty of water and a good detergent. Rinse multiple times to ensure no lye residue remains. Dispose of any lye containers or unused lye safely according to local hazardous waste disposal guidelines.

Although working with lye presents challenges, the rewards of creating your own natural soaps are invaluable. With proper precautions, you can handle lye safely and continue to explore the myriad of possibilities in soapmaking. Empower yourself with knowledge and practice, and you'll find that lye safety becomes second nature, allowing you to focus on crafting beautiful, natural soaps that are kinder to your skin and the environment. Remember, every master soapmaker once stood where you are now, equipped with caution, respect for lye, and a passion for creation.

The Role of Water in Soapmaking

Water is crucial yet often underrated by many soapmaking enthusiasts. Water acts as the solvent that dissolves lye (sodium hydroxide), enabling the essential chemical reaction known as saponification, where oils and fats are transformed into soap. Without water, this fundamental process wouldn't occur, and you'd be left with a mixture of unused oils and lye crystals. The choice of water and how you handle it can significantly impact your final product, from the texture and hardness of your soap to its curing time and shelf life.

To start, let's talk about the various types of water commonly used in soapmaking and their advantages. Most soapmakers prefer distilled water because it is free from minerals and impurities. Minerals in hard water can react with lye and oils, resulting in an inconsistent soap. Softened water is also acceptable and can be a good option if distilled water is unavailable. Some advanced soapmakers even experiment with rainwater or herbal infusions, adding another dimension to their artisanal creations. However, these options come with their own set of challenges, like potential contamination or unpredictable chemical reactions.

Once you've selected your water, the next step is combining it with lye. This stage of soapmaking requires extreme caution due to the caustic nature of the lye solution. Always add lye to water, never the other way around, to prevent dangerous splashes that can cause severe burns. Personal protective equipment like gloves, goggles, and long sleeves should be non-negotiable during this phase. When lye and water are mixed, the solution can reach temperatures as high as 200 degrees Fahrenheit, so ensure that you use heat-resistant, non-reactive containers like stainless steel or heavy-duty plastic.

The temperature of the lye solution and your oils when they're combined is another critical detail. Some soapmakers prefer what's known as the "room temperature method," where both the lye solution and oils are cooled to room temperature before being mixed. This approach can give you more time to work with your soap batter and create intricate designs. Others might combine them at higher temperatures to speed up the saponification process, which can be particularly useful in cold environments. Either way, having an accurate thermometer handy is essential to ensure you hit the right temperatures for your specific recipe.

Adding your lye solution to your oils is where you'll notice the transformation beginning. The water helps the lye penetrate and break down the fats and oils, allowing them to recombine as soap. Initially, the mixture will be thin, but as you stir or use a stick blender, it will start to thicken. This is what's known as "trace," a stage where the mixture has emulsified enough that droplets or trails will remain on the surface for a few seconds. Reaching this stage is crucial before any additives like fragrance oils, colorants, or exfoliants are introduced.

Water also plays a key role in the curing process, which is essential for creating a bar of soap that's mild and long-lasting. After you've poured your soap batter into molds and allowed it to set, typically for 24 to 48 hours, the next step is removing it and letting it cure. During this curing stage, soap needs to dry out and harden, a process where water gradually evaporates from the bars. The length of the curing time can vary widely but usually lasts between four to six weeks. This slow evaporation not only hardens the bar, making it last longer but also improves its lather and overall quality.

For those interested in experimenting, water offers ample room for creativity. Herbal infusions, teas, and even fruit juices can replace plain distilled water to add subtle scents, colors, and therapeutic benefits to your soap. For example, using chamomile tea instead of water can produce a soothing soap ideal for sensitive skin. Green tea, loaded with antioxidants, can be a great addition for more rejuvenating and refreshing bars. However, be mindful of the pH levels and potential for spoilage when using alternate liquids.

It's also worth noting that less water can lead to a faster tracing and harder bars, but it can be trickier to work with. This approach, known as water discounting, is often used by experienced soapmakers who are looking to speed up curing times and create a harder, longer-lasting bar. However, reduced water can also make the batter thicker and harder to pour, requiring rapid and precise work. It's a balancing act that demands a good understanding of your ingredients and the desired outcome.

Finally, consider the ecological aspect of your water use. Water conservation is increasingly critical, even in the artistry of soapmaking. Simple steps such as using only the amount of water needed, reusing rinse water for cleaning equipment, or opting for rainwater can make your soapmaking practice more sustainable. Conscious water usage is a small but impactful way to contribute to a more sustainable future while crafting beautiful, natural soaps.

In summary, water is far more than just another ingredient in the soapmaking process. It acts as a catalyst for saponification, dictates the quality of the final product, and offers a canvas for creative experimentation. By understanding the role of water and how to manipulate it effectively, you'll gain greater control over your soapmaking endeavors and produce creations that are not only beautiful but functional and eco-friendly.

Chapter 4:
Designing Your Soap Recipes

Creating your own unique soap recipes is where the magic truly begins. As a soapmaker, this is your canvas—an opportunity to combine creativity with science to craft personal masterpieces. Start by understanding the vital balance between lye and oils, adhering to safe ratios that ensure a skin-friendly product. Beyond basic calculations, dive into the fun realm of customizing soap properties by selecting specific oils, butters, and additives that imbue your bars with desired characteristics like lather, creaminess, or hardness. Remember, there's an art to this—they don't call it soapmaking for nothing. Keep experimenting with different combinations and be open to happy accidents; sometimes the most unexpected tweaks can yield extraordinary results. With each batch, you'll refine your techniques and develop an intuitive sense for what works best, empowering you to elevate your soap to a whole new level of artistry and function.

Calculating Lye and Oil Ratios ...

When it comes to crafting the perfect bar of soap, understanding how to calculate lye and oil ratios is pivotal. This step marks the harmonious marriage of science and art, resulting in a product that's both luxurious and functional. The ratio between lye and oils determines not just the hardness of your soap but also its moisturizing properties, its lather, and even how long it takes to cure. Let's dive into this essential aspect of soapmaking.

First things first, every oil has a specific saponification value (often shortened to 'SAP value'). This value tells you the amount of lye necessary to completely saponify that particular oil. Whether you're using olive oil, coconut oil, or shea butter, each will require a different amount of lye to convert it into soap. SAP values are usually provided in the form of a range, and it's crucial to choose a reliable source for these values because even small discrepancies can impact your soap's quality.

To make the calculation process straightforward, soapmakers often rely on what's called a 'lye calculator.' These online tools simplify the entire process by taking in your oil choices and quantities, then outputting the exact amount of lye required for the batch. However, having a fundamental understanding of what's happening behind the scenes will make you a more versatile and confident soapmaker.

Let's break down a basic formula: an oil's weight multiplied by its SAP value equals the amount of lye needed. For instance, if you're using 500 grams of olive oil (with a SAP value of 0.134), you'll need 67 grams of lye to saponify that oil completely. Each type of oil you include in your recipe will require you to make this calculation and then sum the lye amounts to get the total lye needed for your soap batch.

While the primary formula is straightforward, there's an art to balancing these ratios to create a bar of soap that's both cleansing and moisturizing. This is where the terms 'superfatting' and 'lye discount' come into play. Superfatting is the process of leaving some oils unsaponified, providing extra emollience to the finished soap. Typically, soapmakers will discount the total lye amount by 5-7% to ensure that some oils remain free-floating in the soap. This provides a moisturizing property, making the soap gentler on the skin.

Accuracy in measuring your lye and oils can't be overstated. Inaccurate measurements can lead to lye-heavy soaps, which are harsh and potentially skin-irritating, or overly oily soaps that may not lather well and could go rancid faster. Always use a digital scale, ensuring precision down to the gram for smaller batches and the tenth of a gram for larger ones.

Another important factor to consider is the type of water used in soapmaking. Distilled water is highly recommended because it doesn't contain minerals or impurities that could react unpredictably with lye. The amount of water you use typically ranges from 25% to 38% of the oil weight, with experienced soapmakers adjusting this based on the specific recipe and environmental conditions.

Balancing the oils in your recipe is equally crucial. Different oils contribute different properties to your soap. For instance, coconut oil adds cleansing power and hardness but can be drying. Olive oil, on the other hand, is excellent for moisturizing but leads to a softer bar. A well-balanced recipe often includes a combination of a few hard oils and some soft oils to achieve the ideal soap texture. Common hard oils include coconut oil, palm oil, and tallow. Common soft oils are olive oil, sunflower oil, and sweet almond oil.

You might wonder how to decide the amounts of each type of oil in your recipes. Many new soapmakers find it helpful to start with established recipes and gradually tweak them to better understand how each oil affects the final product. For custom formulas, you can aim for a composition like this: 30% hard oils for hardness and stability, 30% conditioning oils for moisturizing properties, and 40% oils proportionally divided depending on the specific traits you want in your soap (like lather or long-lasting bars).

When designing a recipe, consider what you want in your final product. Do you want a soap that's more moisturizing? Focus more on high-oleic oils like olive and sweet almond oil. Looking for a rich, stable lather? Coconut and castor oils are excellent choices.

Highlighting this balance for intentional benefits ensures that your end product will meet your personal or business needs.

As a soapmaker, you'll also have to adjust your lye and oil ratios based on seasonal or environmental changes. High humidity can affect your soap curing time and even how your lye solution behaves. In winter, some oils like coconut oil may solidify, requiring a bit of warming before you can measure and use them effectively. These subtle adjustments, while not fundamentally altering your ratios, do influence your overall soapmaking process.

But it's not just about the ratios—technique matters too. Always add your lye to water, never the other way around. This step is vital for safety and for ensuring that the lye solution dissolves completely. Using heat-resistant plastic or stainless steel containers is also crucial, as these materials won't react with lye. High-quality thermometers help you keep track of temperature, ensuring that both your oils and lye solution are within the optimal range (usually between 100-130°F) before mixing them together.

Finally, don't underestimate the value of testing and patience. Always test your soap's pH level once it's cured to ensure it falls within the safe range of 7 to 10. It's also wise to take notes on every batch you make. Record your ratios, the quantities used, and any observations during the soapmaking and curing process, so you can refine and perfect your recipes over time.

Arming yourself with the knowledge of how to calculate lye and oil ratios, combined with a bit of hands-on practice, will set you on the path to mastering soapmaking. It's in these details where true artistry and science meet, enabling you to create bars of soap that are not only functional but also filled with the care and precision that make homemade products so deeply satisfying.

Customizing Soap Properties

Customizing soap's properties is a delightful aspect of soapmaking that can truly elevate your creations to new heights. Once you've mastered the basics, you can begin to experiment with various ingredients to tailor the properties of your soap to meet your specific needs or preferences. This not only allows you to create unique products but also enables you to craft soaps that cater to different skin types, seasons, and personal tastes. Customizing involves tweaking the formula by adjusting oils, superfatting levels, essential oils, and additives.

First, consider the types of oils and butters you use. Each oil and fat contributes its own unique properties to the soap. For example, olive oil is renowned for its moisturizing qualities and is gentle on the skin, making it an ideal choice for sensitive skin soaps. On the other hand, coconut oil is known for creating a hard bar with a bubbly lather, though using too much can make the soap drying. Balancing these oils properly is key to getting the desired hardness, moisturizing properties, and lather.

Shea butter and cocoa butter introduce rich moisturizing characteristics and add a luxurious feel to the soap. Adding them in higher percentages can result in a creamier texture and increased conditioning effects. However, it's essential to maintain a balance; too much of these can make the soap too soft or greasy. Each batch of soap acts as a blank canvas where you can mix and match these ingredients to achieve a distinct profile.

Another important aspect to customize is the superfatting level. Superfatting refers to the amount of free oils left in the soap that haven't been saponified. These extra oils add moisturizing properties and richness to the final product. Typically, a superfat level between 3-8% is used in most recipes. Increasing the superfat level will make your soap more conditioning but might slightly reduce its lathering ability.

Essential oils aren't just about how your soap smells; they bring along various beneficial properties. Tea tree oil, for instance, is excellent for acne-prone skin due to its antibacterial properties. Lavender essential oil can be calming for both the skin and mind, making it great for an evening bath soap. Eucalyptus essential oil adds a refreshing scent and can help clear sinuses, turning your morning shower into an invigorating experience. When selecting essential oils, consider both their olfactory and therapeutic effects to enhance your soap's utility.

Adding botanical ingredients is another fun and functional way to customize your soap. Dried herbs, like chamomile and calendula, can provide soothing and anti-inflammatory properties. These botanicals can be integrated into the soap in various forms, such as infused oils or as whole dried flowers within the soap itself. For instance, you can make a chamomile-infused oil by steeping dried chamomile flowers in a carrier oil, then using this infused oil as part of your soap recipe.

Exfoliants are also an excellent addition for customizing your soap. Ground oats, coffee grounds, and poppy seeds can add different levels of exfoliation, from gentle to more robust scrubbing effects. Such exfoliants not only enhance the texture of your soap but also add another layer of functionality. For example, coffee grounds are great for removing odors and can be excellent in kitchen soaps, while poppy seeds provide a gentle scrub suitable for face and body bars. Incorporating these elements thoughtfully can result in soaps that cleanse, exfoliate, and leave your skin feeling rejuvenated.

Don't overlook the importance of the liquids used in your soapmaking. While water is the most common base, using alternative liquids can infuse your soap with unique qualities. Goat milk, for instance, adds creaminess and extra moisturization due to its high-fat content. You can also use herbal teas, hydrosols, or even fruit and vegetable juices to impart additional nutrients and subtle fragrances into your soap. Keep in mind that these liquids can alter the behavior of your lye solution, so always test in small batches first.

The pH level of your soap is a critical property to dial in. Most good-quality soap falls in the pH range of 8-10, slightly alkaline. Testing and adjusting your soap's pH can make it milder and more suitable for sensitive skin. This involves measuring the pH with a reliable pH strip or digital meter and adjusting your ingredients accordingly to achieve the desired level.

Customizing your soap properties isn't only about aesthetics and feel but also about ensuring the longevity and performance of your soap. Adding a small amount of sodium lactate or salt can harden your soap, making it last longer and perform well under shower conditions. These additives can be particularly beneficial if you reside in a humid environment where soap tends to become mushy.

Let's not forget the visual appeal of your customized soap. Natural colorants such as clays and plant-based powders can introduce a range of shades from earthy tones to vibrant hues. Red Moroccan clay can provide a rich, warm color along with excellent cleansing properties, while spirulina will lend your soap a beautiful green shade and bring in antioxidants and vitamins. These colorants can help you create visually striking soaps that also cater to your skin's needs.

Once you have your recipe figured out, record each detail meticulously. Documenting your process will help you replicate successful batches and tweak the less successful ones. Customizing soap properties is both an art and a science, requiring careful observation, experimentation, and adjustment. This practice is not only rewarding but also adds a personal touch to every bar of soap you create, making each one a work of art and function.

Tailoring the properties of your soap enhances its benefits while also showcasing your creativity. Each ingredient contributes to the overall feel, performance, and appearance of the final product. So, by understanding and manipulating these components, you can produce soaps that are truly unique and cater to specific needs, from therapeutic benefits to aesthetic appeal. In the end, the customization of soap properties is a journey of discovery and creativity that keeps the craft engaging and endlessly rewarding.

Recipe Formulation Tips and Tricks

The joy of soapmaking lies not just in the act of creation, but in the freedom to tailor each bar to your unique needs and preferences. In this section, we'll delve into some of the most valuable tips and tricks to help you on your way to formulating your own soap recipes. Whether you're dreaming up your very first batch or looking to elevate your soapmaking skills, these insights will provide a robust foundation for your soapy creations.

First and foremost, understanding the primary role of each ingredient in your soap recipe is key to effective formulation. Oils and butters each bring their own unique properties to soap. For instance, olive oil is known for its moisturizing qualities, while coconut oil provides a great lather. When combining different oils and butters, aim to balance hardness, lather, and conditioning properties for a well-rounded bar of soap.

One of the best tricks in the realm of soapmaking is to master the art of balancing your oils. A common starting formula is to use 30% olive oil, 30% coconut oil, 30% palm oil or a palm-free substitute, and 10% castor oil. This balanced approach ensures you get the right mix of cleansing, moisturizing, and bubbly lather. Feel free to adjust the percentages slightly to suit your preferences or the needs of your skin.

An essential part of tweaking your soap recipe is the concept of superfatting. Superfatting is essentially adding extra fat to the recipe to enrich the soap with moisturizing properties. The usual range for superfatting is between 5-8%. If you're making soap for dry or sensitive skin, you might want to aim for the higher end of that range. On the other hand, soaps designed for oily skin might benefit from a lower superfat percentage.

Next, let's talk additives. Adding herbs and botanicals to your soap not only boosts its aesthetic appeal but also imparts additional skin benefits. However, it's crucial to properly prepare these additives to avoid any mishaps. Drying herbs thoroughly prevents mold and decomposition within the soap. Finely powdered, coarsely ground, or kept whole, the form of the herb can dramatically change the effect within the final product.

When it comes to incorporating essential oils, less is often more. Essential oils are potent, and overuse can lead to skin irritation. Generally, a usage rate of 0.5-1 ounce of essential oil per pound of soap is adequate. Always refer to an essential oil safety chart to ensure that you are using safe dilution rates. A well-blended essential oil combination not only smells incredible but can also offer aromatherapeutic benefits.

Consider also the temperature at which you mix your oils and lye solution. Keeping both your oils and lye at a similar temperature, generally around 100-110°F, ensures a smoother mixing process and can prevent issues like false trace. False trace occurs when the soap batter thickens prematurely due to temperature differences, leading to an uneven or failed batch.

Another nifty trick is to use a soap calculator. Soap calculators are invaluable tools for both novice and experienced soap makers. They help you to understand the properties your finished product will have and ensure that you are using the correct amount of lye for your chosen oils. These calculators can also predict lather quality, bar hardness, and the overall conditioning effects of your ingredients.

For those eager to add natural colorants, keep in mind that they often behave differently from synthetic dyes. Natural colorants like clays, plant-based powders, and infused oils can add beautiful hues but need to be used with understanding of their quirks. For instance, different types of clay can give you a spectrum of earthy colors, but their high absorbency can also affect the final texture of your soap. Testing small batches is the best way to understand how a new additive will perform.

Playing with textures and visual elements is another exciting part of recipe formulation. Techniques such as layering, swirling, and embedding can transform the look of your soaps. Begin by mastering simple layers or swirling methods before moving on to more complex designs. Remember, there's no right or wrong way—only endless possibilities to explore and enjoy.

Tracking your results is an oft-overlooked but critical component in recipe development. Maintain a dedicated notebook or digital log for each batch you make, noting down specifics such as temperature, ingredient ratios, and any additives used. Document the final results, including texture, scent, and how the soap feels on your skin. This record will serve as a valuable reference, making it easier to repeat successful recipes and tweak those that need improvement.

One more valuable piece of advice is to always keep sustainability in mind. Using organic or responsibly sourced ingredients not only benefits your skin but also supports environmentally friendly practices. Palm oil, for instance, is a controversial ingredient due to its environmental impact. If you choose to use it, look for sustainable sources certified by organizations like the Roundtable on Sustainable Palm Oil (RSPO). Better yet, explore alternatives like babassu oil or cocoa butter, which can offer similar properties without the ecological concerns.

Last but not least, embrace the spirit of experimentation. Don't be afraid to try out new ingredients or techniques, even if the results are not what you expected. Each batch of soap you make teaches you something new, and it's through these mini discoveries that truly unique and personalized soaps are born.

In conclusion, there are myriad ways to approach the art of soap recipe formulation. From understanding your ingredients and mastering basic formulas to incorporating beneficial additives and colorants, each element adds another layer of depth to your creations. Keep in mind the balance of oils, the importance of superfatting, the magic of natural additives, and the joy of experimenting. By following these tips and tricks, you're well on your way to crafting beautifully unique soaps that reflect your personal style and suit your specific needs.

Happy soaping!

Chapter 5:
The Melt and Pour Method

The Melt and Pour Method is a fantastic entry point for both novice and seasoned soapmakers looking to unleash their creativity without the complexities of cold or hot process soapmaking. This straightforward technique involves melting a pre-made soap base and incorporating your chosen additives, such as herbs, essential oils, colorants, and textures, before pouring the mixture into molds. It's incredibly versatile and offers quick results, making it perfect for experimenting with intricate designs, layered effects, and unique textures. Moreover, the method is highly customizable, enabling you to tailor each batch to your aesthetic and functional preferences while sidestepping the need to handle lye directly. Whether you're crafting for personal use, gifting, or selling at markets, Melt and Pour allows for a delightful blend of simplicity and sophistication, ensuring that every soaping session becomes a rewarding creative escape.

Getting Started with Melt and Pour

This is like embarking on an exciting adventure. The melt and pour method offers the perfect gateway for beginners and even seasoned soapmakers looking for a quick, creative fix. Unlike the cold or hot process methods, melt and pour soap doesn't require handling lye, making it a safe and simple process. Whether you're crafting soaps for personal use, gifts, or a small business, this method provides a foundation that's both fun and filled with endless possibilities.

Essential Soaps

The first thing you'll need is a good-quality melt and pour soap base. These bases come pre-made, often with ingredients like glycerin, goat milk, or shea butter, and they can be found online or at local craft stores. What makes them so versatile is their transparency and ease of melting down, allowing you to customize with colors, fragrances, and additives without the complexities of traditional soapmaking.

Melt and pour soap bases are available in various types, each offering unique properties. A clear glycerin base is perfect for showcasing embedded objects or creating vibrant, transparent bars. If you prefer a more moisturizing soap, opt for a goat milk or shea butter base. Each type has its own melt point and consistency, so it's worth experimenting to find what works best for you.

Once you've chosen your soap base, you'll need a few other essentials: a heat-safe container for melting, a microwave or double boiler, soap molds, and stirring utensils. It's important to gather all your ingredients and equipment before you get started. Preparation is key to a smooth and enjoyable soapmaking session.

Melting the soap base is the next step. You can do this either in a microwave or a double boiler. If you're using a microwave, heat the soap base in short bursts of 15-30 seconds, stirring in between to ensure even melting. If you prefer a double boiler, place your heat-safe container in a pot of gently simmering water. Stir frequently to avoid any hotspots.

Once your soap base is melted, it's time to get creative. Add fragrances, essential oils, colorants, and any other additives you desire. This is where you can really let your creativity shine. Whether it's a vibrant hue from natural colorants or a calming lavender scent from essential oils, the possibilities are virtually endless.

When adding fragrances or essential oils, remember that a little goes a long way. Typically, about 1-2 teaspoons per pound of soap base is sufficient. Be sure to mix thoroughly to ensure the scent is evenly distributed throughout the soap. It's also the perfect time to incorporate herbs, exfoliants, or other textured elements. Just sprinkle them in and stir gently to distribute them evenly.

Color can be added using liquid soap dyes, mica powders, or even natural ingredients such as turmeric or activated charcoal. If you're using powders, make sure to mix them with a small amount of the melted soap base first to avoid clumping. Always blend thoroughly to achieve an even color.

Now that your soap mixture is ready, it's time to pour it into molds. Silicone molds are a great choice as they come in various shapes and sizes and make unmolding the soap easy. Slowly pour the soap mixture to minimize bubbles, and gently tap the mold on a flat surface to release any trapped air. If bubbles persist, you can spritz the surface with a bit of rubbing alcohol to dissolve them.

Allow the soap to cool and harden. This can take a few hours at room temperature. If you're in a hurry, you can place the molds in the refrigerator, but avoid the freezer as it can cause the soap to become too brittle.

Once the soap is fully hardened, gently remove it from the molds. If you used intricate designs, take your time to avoid breaking any delicate parts. Your handcrafted soap is now ready for use! However, if you added any rough herbs or textures, a curing period of a few days might be beneficial to allow them to soften and meld with the soap base.

One of the great things about melt and pour soap is its instant gratification. There's no curing time required, meaning you can use your soap right away. This makes it an excellent choice for last-minute gifts or quick inventory for your craft market stall.

While melt and pour is simpler than other methods, don't underestimate its potential. You can layer different colors, embed objects, or even create soap with intricate details that are sure to impress. The ease of this method allows you to focus more on the artistic and sensory aspects of soapmaking.

For those who love experimenting, the melt and pour method is versatile enough to allow you to try new techniques without committing a lot of time and resources. Make layered soaps by pouring one layer, letting it harden, and then adding another. Add a touch of luxury with specialty oils or butters to the melted soap base. The opportunities for customization are boundless.

This method also lends itself well to business ventures. If you're planning to sell your soaps, the melt and pour technique is an efficient way to build an impressive inventory quickly. Plus, the visually stunning soaps you create can easily stand out in a crowded market. Don't forget to label your soaps with all ingredients, which is particularly essential if you're selling at markets or online.

In summary, the melt and pour method is your invitation to start soapmaking with ease and creativity. It's accessible, fun, and offers endless potential for customization. Whether you're a beginner or an experienced soapmaker, the simplicity and versatility of melt and pour soap will keep you coming back for more. So gather your supplies, ignite your imagination, and let your soapmaking journey begin!

Creative Designs and Techniques

This opens up a world of possibilities for soapmaking enthusiasts, allowing them to transform basic soap bars into works of art. The melt and pour method, in particular, lends itself beautifully to creativity due to its simplicity and flexibility. Whether you're making soap for personal use or to sell, adding an artistic touch can make your soap stand out. Let's dive into some inspiring and achievable creative designs and techniques just for melt and pour soapmaking.

One of the easiest ways to create visually stunning soaps is through layering. Layering involves pouring different soap bases in stages, allowing each layer to set partially before adding the next. The result is a visually arresting soap bar with distinct, colorful layers. To add an extra dimension, you might even embed small objects or chunks of contrasting soap in between the layers. When slicing through, you'll unveil a hidden surprise, captivating both you and anyone you gift or sell the soap to.

Another popular technique is embedding, where pre-made soap pieces are inserted into the soap base. This can be anything from small soap embeds shaped like hearts, stars, or fruit slices. The embedded pieces not only create lovely designs, but they also add a playful element to the soap. Imagine a child's delight upon discovering a dinosaur or unicorn hidden within their soap! To achieve this, melt your base soap, pour a thin layer into your mold, place the embeds carefully, and then pour the remaining base. This ensures the embeds stay put and don't float to the top.

Texture is another creative dimension you can explore. By incorporating materials like oatmeal, coffee grounds, or poppy seeds, you can create soaps that are not only visually interesting but also have a pleasantly exfoliating texture. Experiment with different textures to find combinations that are visually appealing and functional, offering delightful scrubbing sensations while using the soap. Imagine a soap bar with the calming scent of lavender and the gentle exfoliation of ground almonds—both relaxing and invigorating!

Swirling techniques offer another layer of artistic expression. Swirls can be achieved by pouring different colored soap bases simultaneously and using a tool to create patterns. While this may sound intricate, starting with simple swirls using a skewer or spoon can yield stunning results. Advanced techniques like the "in-the-pot swirl" can produce intricate designs that look like they took hours to craft. The trick lies in understanding how different colors and patterns interact once they set. A soap with blue and white swirls, for example, can invoke the calming allure of ocean waves.

Adding botanicals such as dried flowers and herbs not only enhances the aesthetic appeal of your soap but also its functionality. Imagine crafting soaps with petals of chamomile or rose, offering both visual beauty and therapeutic properties. When adding botanicals, make sure they are dried completely to prevent mold formation. Additionally, placing them on the top of the soap rather than throughout the entire bar can maintain the soap's integrity and prolong its shelf life.

For those seeking an extra challenge, try creating a marbled effect. Marbling is similar to swirling but requires more precision. Here, you'll pour layers of different colored soap base and use a tool to create intricate, vein-like patterns. This technique results in soaps that are as unique as natural gemstones. To achieve the best results, work with a firmer soap base, as this will help to hold the design better and prevent colors from blending too much.

Don't overlook the power of molds in adding uniqueness to your soaps. While basic rectangular molds are practical, there are myriad shapes and designs available that can add charm and character to your soap bars. From floral shapes to intricate patterns resembling lace, the right mold can turn an ordinary soap bar into a masterpiece. Silicone molds are especially versatile, offering ease of use and a high level of detail.

Transparency can be a game-changer in soap artistry. Using clear soap bases allows you to create beautiful transparent soaps, perfect for showcasing embeds or intricate swirls. A transparent soap with embedded botanicals like marigold petals or mint leaves can be both visually striking and refreshing to use. The transparency draws attention to the details within, making every wash a visually engaging experience.

If you're feeling festive, holiday-themed soaps can be a delightful endeavor. Whether it's gingerbread men for Christmas or heart shapes for Valentine's Day, themed soaps allow for creative exploration tied to celebrations. Adding scents that evoke the festivities, such as peppermint for Christmas or rose for Valentine's, can enhance the overall experience, making your themed soaps the perfect seasonal gift.

Gradient pours, also known as ombre techniques, provide a way to transition colors gradually within your soap bars. This is accomplished by pouring each layer with a slightly different shade of colorant and allowing it to set partially before adding the next layer. The result is a smooth, gradient transition of colors that can be striking to the eye. Think of a bar that transitions from deep ocean blue to a light sky blue. The visual appeal of this technique can captivate anyone who lays eyes on your soap creations.

Layered soaps aren't limited to horizontal layers. Vertical layering can create stripes or geometric designs that are equally captivating. You can achieve this by dividing your mold and pouring different colored bases side by side or using dividers. Experiment with varying widths of layers to create unique, eye-catching designs that tell a story of meticulous craftsmanship.

Consider the use of mica powders for a shimmering, metallic effect in your soaps. These powders are available in a variety of colors and can be mixed into your soap base to give a gleaming finish. When using mica, make sure to disperse it well to avoid clumping. A bar with a subtle gold or silver shimmer can be especially elegant, making it an excellent choice for special occasions or gifts.

Don't shy away from experimenting with dye effects. Liquid dyes and lab colors can be blended to create custom shades. Try using a combination of different dyes to develop a signature soap color that stands out. Whether it's a bold and vibrant hue or a subtle pastel, color variation can make your soap bars unique and instantly recognizable.

Last but not least, the use of essential oils isn't just for aroma; they can influence the final aesthetic. Citrus oils can tint your soap with subtle shades of orange or yellow, whereas mint oils might give a hint of green. By carefully selecting and blending essential oils, you can create a cohesive sensory experience where the look and scent of the soap work in harmony.

Whether you're just starting or have been making soaps for years, there's always a new technique to master or a new design to try. Soapmaking is an art and, like all art forms, it thrives on experimentation and creativity. So, keep experimenting, keep creating, and let your imagination guide you to new soapy heights!

Adding Herbs, Colorants, and Textures

This is where the magic happens and your soap creations really come to life. Here's where you can indulge your creativity and experiment with various natural ingredients to make your soap not only functional but also a visual and sensory delight. When using the melt and pour method, you have the perfect canvas to incorporate an array of herbs, natural colorants, and textures that can transform your soaps into intricate works of art with beneficial properties.

Herbs offer not only aesthetic appeal but also therapeutic benefits. Lavender, chamomile, and calendula are some of the popular choices that can be used either dried or infused into oils. Lavender adds a gentle exfoliating texture and a calming scent that's perfect for relaxation. Chamomile is soothing and gentle, making it an excellent choice for soaps meant for sensitive skin. Calendula petals, with their vibrant yellow color, add a touch of brightness and have anti-inflammatory properties. When adding dried herbs to your soap base, ensure they are finely ground if you prefer a smoother texture. Coarser particles can sometimes be abrasive. Additionally, some herbs may change color when they interact with the soap base, so it might be wise to do a small test batch first.

Colorants are another exciting element to play with. Natural colorants derived from plants, clays, and other minerals can result in soft, earthy tones or vibrant hues. Spirulina powder gives a beautiful green shade and is rich in antioxidants. Activated charcoal provides a stunning black color and is known for its detoxifying properties. Turmeric, with its warm yellow-orange hue, not only colors your soap but also imparts anti-inflammatory benefits. Clays like kaolin, French green, or rhassoul not only add color but also beneficial cleansing and skin-purifying properties. Each colorant has unique interactions with the soap base—some might bleed or fade over time, so it's essential to understand their characteristics through experimentation.

Textures turn your soap into a tactile experience, offering scrubbing and polishing effects. Oatmeal is a popular additive that's gentle enough for face and body scrubs, offering a soothing feel suitable for sensitive skin. Coffee grounds provide a more intense exfoliation, perfect for scrubbing away dead skin cells and invigorating your senses with a subtle coffee aroma. Seeds like poppy, raspberry, or strawberry not only give a speckled look but also offer moderate exfoliation. When you're incorporating textures, it's all about balance. Too much can make the soap feel overly abrasive, while too little might not provide the tactile experience you're aiming for.

Combining these elements properly can be a creative endeavor that's both enjoyable and rewarding. Begin by selecting a melt and pour soap base according to your preference—transparent or opaque bases work well. Heat the base gently until it's fully melted. This is your blank canvas, ready for your imaginative additions. For herbs, aim to use about one tablespoon per pound of soap base. Sprinkle them in post-melting and stir gently to distribute them evenly. If you're using colorants, start with small amounts—as little as 1/4 teaspoon per pound of soap base—then adjust to your desired shade. For a more vibrant color, you may need to increase the amount, keeping in mind that some natural colorants can stain skin or surfaces if used in excess.

Textures can be added similarly, post-melting. For oatmeal or other fine grains, about one tablespoon per pound of soap base will offer a smooth scrubbing action. Coarser additives like coffee grounds or seeds may only require one to two teaspoons per pound depending on your desired level of exfoliation. Again, stir gently to integrate them into the base completely. To prevent settling of heavier particles, a quick stir just before pouring the soap into molds can help distribute them evenly.

Layering and swirling are techniques that can add even more complexity and interest to your soap designs. Begin by pouring a base layer of melted soap and allowing it to set slightly. Add an herb or colorant to a portion of your remaining soap and pour it over the base layer. You can create multiple layers this way. Swirling can be achieved by adding your colorant to a portion of the soap, then pouring it into the mold and using a skewer or spoon to create swirls. This not only mixes the colors in appealing patterns but also allows you to incorporate different textures at different layers.

Incorporating these elements is also about balance and knowing the interactions between different herbs, colorants, and textures with your soap base. As these are natural ingredients, their properties might change over time. Herbs might lose color, some colorants might fade or change under different lighting conditions, and textures might settle differently. Don't hesitate to experiment with small batches to see their long-term effects and interactions. Documenting your recipes and techniques can be incredibly helpful in fine-tuning future batches.

Beyond the aesthetic and sensory appeal, there's a personal satisfaction that comes from crafting soaps that reflect your style and preferences. Handmade soaps with herbs, natural colorants, and textures are not only beautiful and beneficial but also demonstrate a commitment to natural and eco-friendly practices. Each bar is unique, a testament to the careful thought and creativity you've invested in its making.

This journey of adding herbs, colorants, and textures to your soaps is a continuous learning process. With each batch, you'll discover new combinations and techniques that enhance the soapmaking experience. It's a delightful intersection of science and art, one that invites you to explore and innovate. So go ahead, open those jars of vibrant powders and delicate petals, and let your imagination guide you to create extraordinary soaps that are as wonderful to use as they are to behold.

Chapter 6:
Cold Process Soapmaking

Cold process soapmaking stands as the quintessential method for crafting natural, artisan soaps right at home. This traditional technique, which relies on saponification—the chemical reaction between oils and lye—allows for endless customization and creativity. For those who relish a hands-on approach, cold process opens the door to a world where you control every ingredient, from luxurious oils and butters to the enchanting aromas of essential oils. Here, patience becomes your ally as the soap cures over four to six weeks, transforming into a bar that's as gentle on the skin as it is rich in character. Whether you're layering textures, swirling vibrant patterns, or just enjoying the meditative rhythm of stirring your mixture, this chapter will guide you through the step-by-step process, igniting both inspiration and confidence to create your very own soap masterpieces.

Step-by-Step Guide to Cold Process

Soapmaking is a rewarding and thorough method to create your soaps from scratch. Though it requires a bit of patience and precision, the end result is a richly textured soap with endless customization options. Let's dive into the steps to get you started on this classic soapmaking technique.

First and foremost, gather all your essential ingredients and equipment. You'll need a digital scale, a heat-resistant bowl, a stainless-steel pot, a stick blender, and a mold for your soap. The ingredients include oils or fats, lye (sodium hydroxide), distilled water, and any additives such as essential oils, herbs, or colorants. Ensuring you have everything at arm's length is essential for a seamless process.

Safety is paramount when handling lye. Wear protective gear, including gloves, goggles, and long sleeves. Lye is highly caustic and can cause chemical burns if it comes into contact with skin. Make sure you're working in a well-ventilated area.

Start by preparing your lye solution. Weigh the exact amount of lye needed and slowly add it to your measured water, never the other way around to avoid a volatile reaction. Stir gently until the lye is fully dissolved. The solution will heat up quickly, so set it aside to cool to around 100-120°F.

While the lye solution is cooling, measure out your oils and fats. Common choices include olive oil, coconut oil, and shea butter. Depending on your recipe, you may also include specialized oils for their unique properties. Melt the solid fats and mix them with the liquid oils until the mixture reaches the desired temperature of around 100-120°F.

Once both the lye solution and the oil mixture are within the correct temperature range, it's time to combine them. Slowly pour the lye solution into the oils while stirring continuously. Use your stick blender to blend the mixture until it reaches "trace," a stage where the mixture thickens, and trails form on the surface when the blender is lifted. This can take anywhere from a few minutes to 15 minutes, depending on your oils and the temperature.

Reaching trace is a critical point where you can incorporate your additives. Add your essential oils, colorants, and any herbs you wish to include. Continue blending the mixture to ensure everything is well incorporated.

Pour the mixture into your prepared mold. Tap the mold slightly on the counter to release any air bubbles. Cover the mold with a lid or plastic wrap, and then insulate it with towels to maintain the heat. This is vital for the saponification process, where the oils and lye transform into soap.

Leave your soap in the mold for 24 to 48 hours. After this period, the soap should be firm enough to unmold. Carefully release the soap from the mold and cut it into bars. These bars will still be in their curing stage and need to be placed in a well-ventilated space for about 4 to 6 weeks. During curing, the soap will lose excess moisture and become milder and firmer.

Labeling and storing your cured soap bars are equally important steps. Note the date they were made, and any specific ingredients used, especially if you plan to market them. Store them in a cool, dry place to extend their shelf life.

Throughout this journey, keep detailed notes of your process and experiments. Record observations such as how quickly your soap traced, the final texture, and any changes you might want to make in future batches. This practice not only helps improve your techniques but also ensures consistency if you're producing soap for sale.

The cold process method offers a sense of fulfillment as each step is a direct involvement in crafting a natural, homemade product. With practice, you'll be inspired to experiment further with textures, layers, and intricate designs as described in the subsequent subsection *Creating Texture and Layers*, helping you to elevate your soapmaking skills to new heights.

Creating Texture and Layers

This is where your soapmaking adventure gets an exciting twist. When you're delving into cold process soapmaking, adding texture and layers is akin to painting on a blank canvas, only your medium is creamy soap batter. Whether you're a first-time hobbyist or an experienced artisan, creating intricate designs can take your soap beyond mere cleanliness to pure artistry.

To begin with, the way you pour your soap batter can dramatically affect its final look. If you pour it at a thin trace, the soap layers will tend to blend more, creating softer lines and abstract patterns. Conversely, soap poured at a thick trace will generally keep its layers distinct, allowing for more defined lines and textures. Knowing the behavior of your batter at different trace stages can set you up for spectacular results.

One compelling technique is to use natural exfoliants and herbs right within your layers. For instance, incorporating oatmeal or ground coffee between soap layers not only provides a visually appealing texture but also serves as a gentle exfoliant. Herbs like calendula petals or lavender buds can add color and texture, offering a dual sensory experience of sight and feel.

Color layering is another powerful tool in your design arsenal. By dividing your soap batter into several portions and coloring each one differently, you can layer them one on top of the other. Imagine a lavender and rosemary soap with alternate layers of soft purple and rich green. These color contrasts can make each slice of soap a mini masterpiece. It's essential to plan your color choices carefully, aiming for a harmonious palette that enhances the soap's overall theme and the benefits of its ingredients.

One popular method for creating distinct layers is by using dividers in your mold. These barriers can be made from thin plastic or cardboard. By segmenting your mold, you can pour different colors or textures of soap batter into each section without them mixing prematurely. Once the sections are filled, you remove the dividers, and voila—perfectly crisp, clean layers. Ensure your dividers are the same height as your mold to achieve uniformity.

Essential Soaps

In addition to plain layers, experimenting with textured layers can elevate your soap to the next level. Imagine layers of soap punctuated by embeds—small, shaped pieces of previously cured soap—suspended between layers. These embeds can be simple cubes or sophisticated shapes like hearts, stars, or even leaves. They add intrigue and make each soap bar unique.

Another tactic for an elegant look is mica lines. Mica is a fine, shimmering powder that can be layered between soap batches to create fine, sparkly lines. To accomplish this, pour a thin layer of soap, then disperse a light dusting of mica powder before pouring the next layer. The result is a series of glimmering stripes that catch the light beautifully and add a touch of luxury to your soap.

Don't overlook the visual impact of ombre effects, where one color transitions seamlessly into another. Achieving this requires devotion to the details. Start by pouring your first layer, then gradually mix small quantities of the next color into the soap batter, pouring layer upon layer. Each successive layer should have slightly more of the second color. This technique does take some practice to perfect, but the result is a striking gradient that can wow your customers or gift recipients.

The mantra of creating texture and layers is to "think outside the box." Feel inspired by the world around you—the colors of a sunset, the stratification of geological formations, or the layers of foam in a latte. Translating these everyday wonders into your soap designs can yield a product that's both personal and universally appealing.

For a fun and unexpected twist, try adding a textured top layer. Swirls, peaks, and even intricate patterns can be achieved by manipulating the top layer of your soap with a spatula, skewer, or spoon. Think of this layer as the finishing touch, like icing on a cake. It's where your personality can shine through—adding dimension and visual appeal that makes your soap irresistible.

Another enchanting technique involves embedding loofahs or bamboo charcoal nets between layers. This not only creates texture but also enhances the soap's functionality by adding natural exfoliating properties. Imagine a refreshing peppermint soap with pieces of loofah embedded; each use gently polishes the skin, leaving it feeling revitalized.

A critical aspect when working with layers is patience. Allowing each layer to set up slightly before adding the next reduces the risk of blending. While the wait might feel tedious, the reward of distinct, defined layers is worth the extra time. This is especially true when working with colors that tend to bleed or fragrances that accelerate trace.

Lastly, remember that less can be more. Sometimes, the simplicity of two or three well-coordinated layers can be more striking than a complex multi-layered piece. It's about finding that perfect balance where each layer tells a part of the story, each texture adds a nuance, and together they create a harmonious, beautiful soap. So, don't shy away from experimenting and pushing your creative boundaries.

Swirling and Patterning Techniques

These techniques elevate your cold process soapmaking from simple bars to beautiful, intricate works of art. These techniques are not just about making visually appealing soaps; they're also about mastering the art of timing, temperature control, and understanding your ingredients. Each swirl tells a story, each pattern speaks of your creativity and skill, thus ensuring a unique signature on each batch.

In the world of swirling and patterning, it's all about the pour. The way you pour your soap batter into the mold creates the foundation for your swirls. A "In-The-Pot Swirl," for instance, involves pouring different colors of soap batter directly into one pot, stirring ever so gently, and then pouring this color-mixed mixture into the mold. This technique yields beautiful, varied swirls, almost as if nature herself painted them.

For those looking for more control over their designs, the "Drop Swirl" technique offers a fantastic middle ground. Here, you pour layers of soap batter in different colors into the mold, allowing them to drop and mix in the mold organically. The result is elegant, elongated patterns that mimic the look of natural stone or marbled paper. It's amazing what gravity and a bit of patience can achieve.

Another crowd favorite is the "Tiger Stripe" pattern. This fun and straightforward technique involves alternating thin pours of different colors down the middle of your mold. As you layer them, they create a vivid, stripy design that brings a touch of the wild to your soap bars. What's brilliant about the Tiger Stripe is its versatility; you can use any combination of colors to match the seasons, holidays, or even to evoke specific moods.

On the more complex end, the "Taiwan Swirl" is a technique that challenges your precision and control. To execute a Taiwan Swirl, you need to create perfectly even vertical lines of different colors along the length of your mold, before dragging a skewer or swirling tool through them to create intricate, feathered designs. The result is a visually stunning soap that often leaves you in awe of its fine, lace-like details. Crafting a successful Taiwan Swirl requires a steady hand and a well-traced plan, but the results are more than worth the effort.

"Hanger Swirls" are particularly fun and versatile. For this technique, you'll use a hanger tool or a looped piece of wire to drag through layers of multiple colored soap batters in your mold. By varying your motions—be it figure-eights, curlicues, or simple zig-zags—you can create a range of delightful patterns. The swirling process here is much like painting in three dimensions, as you're drawing not just on the surface but throughout the entire depth of the soap.

If you're interested in structurally distinctive patterns, try the "Peacock Swirl." This technique starts with a base layer of soap in your mold. Then you pour lines of different colors horizontally across the mold's surface. After that, you drag a skewer vertically up and down the length of the soap, followed by a series of horizontal drag motions, all while maintaining equidistance. This effort gives the finished soap the exotic, feathered look reminiscent of a peacock's tail.

Sometimes, the simplicity of a "Chopstick Swirl" can be extraordinarily elegant. With this method, after pouring multiple colors into your mold either in layers or spots, you'll take a chopstick or bamboo skewer and gently swirl through the soap batter in various directions. The beauty of this technique lies in its spontaneity; no two chopstick swirls will ever come out the same. It's a wonderful way to let creativity flow without the rigidity of a predetermined design.

It's important to note that each swirling technique has its own set of challenges and requires a good understanding of trace. Trace is the stage in soapmaking where the batter thickens and can hold patterns. Too thin, and the colors will blend too much; too thick, and it becomes difficult to swirl. Mastering the balance of trace is key to achieving stunning swirling patterns.

Temperature plays a crucial role as well. Cooler temperatures allow for more intricate swirls since the soap batter stays fluid for a longer time. However, working at cooler temperatures requires patience and experience, as it can also slow down the saponification process. On the opposite end, warmer temperatures cause the batter to thicken more quickly, which could be beneficial for certain patterns but limits the time you have to work on your design.

Beyond technique, the choice of colors and additives also influences your swirls and patterns. Micas, oxides, and natural colorants like spirulina and madder root each behave differently in soap. For instance, natural colorants can sometimes morph during saponification due to the high pH, transforming from one hue to another. Understanding these nuances allows you to predict and control the final appearance of your bar.

Pigments that boast stability, such as oxides and ultramarines, generally retain their vibrancy during the soapmaking process. Their predictability can make them easier for beginners to work with, while natural botanicals often offer more muted and earthy tones. Every pigment has a personality, and discovering how each interacts with your soap formula is part of the adventure.

Equally, having the right tools will make your journey smoother. While a simple chopstick and wire hanger can create beautiful designs, investing in swirling tools such as swirling dividers and squeeze bottles can elevate your game. These tools allow more precision in placement and motion, crucial for more intricate patterns like the "Secret Feather Swirl" or "Spiraled Column Swirl."

As you become more comfortable with these techniques, you may start to develop your own signature styles. Combining methods, experimenting with color combinations, and incorporating different additives like glitter or fine grains can open up endless possibilities. The joy truly comes from the experimentation—there are no real mistakes, only lessons and unexpected beauty.

Incorporating herbs and botanicals further expands your creative potential. Imagine a lavender essential oil soap with purple mica swirls, speckled with dried lavender buds. Or a bright citrus bar with orange and yellow swirls, embedded with poppy seeds for a light exfoliation. These not only look stunning but also enhance the sensory experience, making each bar a little piece of functional art.

Swirling and patterning speak directly to the harmony of nature and art. It brings an added dimension to soapmaking, turning each bar into a unique creation. With each new batch, you'll find that the journey isn't just about the soap, but also about expressing yourself, experimenting, and evolving as a soapmaker. Dive in, let your creativity take the reins, and watch as your soapmaking transforms into an artistic expression that both looks beautiful and performs wonderfully.

Chapter 7:
Hot Process Soapmaking

Hot process soapmaking brings a unique and rewarding twist to crafting your own soap, marrying the thrill of creativity with a shorter cure time. Using high heat to speed up saponification, this method allows you to enjoy fully usable soap almost immediately after it cools. It's a favored choice for those who relish both the art and the efficiency it offers. Whether you opt for a trusty crock pot or an oven-safe dish, you'll find this technique infuses a rustic, textured finish to your bars that cold process enthusiasts often admire. The real beauty of hot process lies in its simplicity—you can even add delicate essential oils and herbs at the end without fearing their degradation from lye. This method offers the magic of chemistry right in your kitchen, turning natural ingredients into beautiful, aromatic soaps laden with your personal touch. Ready to dive in? Your soaping adventure awaits!

The Basics of Hot Process

Hot process soapmaking is an exciting, hands-on method that's loved by many for its rustic charm and forgiving nature. For those unfamiliar, the hot process (HP) method utilizes heat to speed up the saponification process, allowing the soap to be ready for use much sooner than cold process soaps. Imagine combining the best of both worlds—the creativity of soapmaking with the gratifying immediacy of a quicker cure time. Let's dive into what makes hot process soapmaking not just straightforward but incredibly rewarding.

In essence, hot process soapmaking involves combining oils and lye, just like in cold process soapmaking, but with an added step: cooking. This cooking phase accelerates saponification—essentially the chemical reaction that turns oils and lye into soap. While cold process soap can take weeks to cure, hot process soap is typically ready to use within a few days. The finished product usually boasts a more rustic, textured appearance which many find endearing and distinctive.

The process begins similarly to other soapmaking methods. Start by weighing and melting your chosen oils. It's crucial to have a well-researched recipe and all your ingredients measured out beforehand. Once the oils are melted and heated to around 120°F-130°F (49°C-54°C), you carefully add your lye solution. Safety first! Always wear gloves and goggles, and work in a well-ventilated area. The initial mixing of oils and lye mirrors cold process soapmaking, but the paths diverge significantly from here on.

For hot process soapmaking, the blended mixture is transferred to a heat source, typically a slow cooker or a double boiler. This is where the "hot" in hot process comes into play. Over the next hour or two, you'll witness the soap transform through several phases. It starts as a thin, pudding-like consistency and then goes through a thick, mashed-potato stage. Eventually, it turns into a more fluid, gel-like substance. This phase is known as the gel phase, a telltale sign that saponification is underway.

Throughout the cooking process, it's essential to stir the mixture periodically. This not only helps distribute the heat but also ensures even saponification. Patience is key here; resist the urge to rush the process. The soap will let you know when it's done—typically, the mixture will become more translucent, and the edges will start to pull away from the sides of your cooking vessel. If you're uncertain, performing a zap test can confirm whether the soap is fully saponified (though always proceed with caution).

Essential Soaps

A significant advantage of the hot process method is the ability to add extra ingredients like colorants, fragrances, and herbs after saponification. This minimizes the risk of these additives reacting with the lye, preserving their potency. Imagine the delight of incorporating delicate essential oils and vibrant botanicals knowing they'll retain their full aromatic and therapeutic benefits. It's a game-changer for those who love to experiment and customize their soap creations.

Once the soap has reached the desired consistency, it's time to mold. The mixture is usually quite thick, so be prepared to work quickly. Spoon or pour the soap into prepared molds, using a spatula to press it into all corners and smooth the top. No need to wait extended periods before removing from the mold, as hot process soap hardens relatively quickly. Within 24 hours, you'll have a solid block of soap ready for cutting and a short cure period before it can be used.

The quick turnaround time from mixing to molding makes hot process soapmaking especially appealing for those looking to produce larger quantities or meet specific deadlines. Small business owners, in particular, find this method beneficial for its efficient process and the premium, handcrafted appeal of the final product.

Moreover, the textured, rustic look of hot process soap offers a unique aesthetic that stands apart from the smoother bars produced through cold process. This look can be further enhanced with creative molds and stamping techniques, adding an artisanal touch that truly makes each bar one-of-a-kind. Picture a bar embedded with specks of herbs or infused with swirls of natural colorants—each bar telling its own unique story.

For those wary of the steep learning curve often associated with soapmaking, hot process offers a forgiving alternative. The cooking phase corrects minor miscalculations in oil or lye ratios that might otherwise spoil a cold process batch. You can think of it as a second chance to get things just right—perfect for beginners still honing their craft or veterans trying out a new recipe.

In terms of sustainability, hot process soapmaking aligns beautifully with eco-friendly practices. The method allows easier incorporation of locally-sourced and seasonal botanicals. Additionally, the reduced curing time means less energy consumption compared to other methods. So, not only are you creating a natural, nourishing product, but you're also contributing to a more sustainable lifestyle.

As you continue on your soapmaking journey, don't shy away from experimenting with hot process soapmaking. The tactile involvement and almost immediate gratification are addictive. Whether you're making soap as a meaningful DIY project, a heartfelt gift, or a small business venture, hot process soap offers a perfect blend of ease, speed, and creative freedom.

Ultimately, mastering the basics of hot process soapmaking opens up a world of possibilities. You'll find yourself more confident in experimenting with new ingredients and designs. Embrace the rustic charm of hot process soap and enjoy the fulfillment of creating something both beautiful and practical with your own hands. It's not just about making soap; it's about crafting a product infused with care, creativity, and a piece of your spirit.

Crock Pot and Oven Methods

These two methods represent traditional yet innovative approaches to hot process soapmaking that modern soap enthusiasts find indispensable. Both techniques allow for more control over the saponification process and can produce a wonderfully rustic, textured bar of soap. Let's dive into the nuances of each method.

The crock pot method, also known as the "crock pot hot process" (CPHP), is particularly beloved for its simplicity and consistency. This approach utilizes the steady, even heat of a slow cooker to speed up saponification. Begin by setting up your soapmaking area with all the necessary equipment: your oils, lye solution, a heat-resistant container, and of course, your crock pot. Pre-warm your crock pot while you prepare your lye and oils, ensuring both reach a similar temperature range around 110°F to 120°F.

Once your ingredients are prepared, pour the oils into the crock pot and add the lye solution in a slow, steady stream, blending continuously. As you mix, you'll notice the soap mixture tracing quickly. Cover the crock pot with its lid and set it to low. The mixture will need to cook for about one to two hours, during which time you should check on it periodically. You will observe the soap go through various stages, transitioning from a mashed potato-like consistency to a gel phase.

The gel phase is a crucial moment in CPHP soapmaking. During this phase, the soap becomes more translucent and gel-like. It's at this stage that the full saponification occurs. You might feel tempted to stir the mixture, but resist this unless absolutely necessary, as it can introduce unwanted air bubbles. When the soap has fully gelled and is no longer opaque, it's ready for any add-ins.

At this point, you can stir in your essential oils, additives like clays, oatmeal, or herbs with ease. The heat retention in the crock pot ensures these elements blend smoothly without the risk of accelerating trace too quickly. After mixing, scoop the hot soap into prepared molds. It's more pliable at this stage, allowing you to create textured tops if desired. Allow the soap to cool and harden for about 24 hours before unmolding it. Unlike cold process soap, which requires a cure time of several weeks, hot process soap made in a crock pot is safe to use much sooner, often within just a few days, since saponification is nearly complete by the end of the cooking process.

Shifting gears, the oven hot process (OHP) method taps into the consistent, expansive heat of a conventional oven, perfect for those larger batches that a crock pot might struggle to contain. Similar to the crock pot method, you'll begin with a mixture of oils and lye, blended to trace. Preheat your oven to around 170°F, an optimal low heat setting for gently cooking your soap without overheating.

Transfer the traced soap mixture into an oven-safe container, preferably a stainless steel pot or an enameled Dutch oven. Cover the container with a lid or aluminum foil. Place the pot in the oven, and let it cook for about one to two hours, checking occasionally to ensure it's moving through its stages properly. You'll notice similar phases as with the crock pot method—first a mashed potato stage, followed by the gel phase where the soap becomes more fluid and gelatinous.

The main benefit of OHP is the ability to make larger batches of soap efficiently. The oven's direct heat can also result in a more consistent gel phase, thanks to the enclosed, uniform environment. Just like with the crock pot method, once the soap has fully gelled and appears translucent, it's ready for add-ins. Carefully remove the hot container from the oven, open the lid, and swiftly but gently mix in any essential oils, colorants, or texturizing ingredients you've prepared. This step can be somewhat tricky as the soap is quite hot, so handle with caution to avoid burns.

After incorporating your chosen additives, pour the soap mixture into molds. Again, you have the opportunity to play with textured tops thanks to the pliability of the hot soap. Leave the soap to cool and harden for at least 24 hours before unmolding. Due to the thorough cooking process, these OHP soaps, like their crock pot counterparts, benefit from a reduced curing time, becoming usable and mild much faster than cold process soaps.

Using the crock pot and oven methods not only speeds up the soapmaking process but also allows for a degree of creativity that's harder to achieve with traditional cold process methods. Both techniques are excellent for those who appreciate a hands-on, immediate approach to soapmaking. The rustic, handcrafted aesthetic achieved through these methods is perfect for small business owners who want to offer unique, artisan products or homesteaders who value making the most of their resources.

The quick turnaround of hot process soaps also aligns well with sustainable practices. Being able to use your soap almost immediately reduces the need for extensive storage space and allows you to make and use soaps in smaller, more manageable batches, cutting down on waste. Plus, the flexibility of adding ingredients post-saponification ensures that the beneficial properties of your essential oils and botanicals are preserved, enhancing the natural qualities of your handmade soap.

So, whether you're seeking speed, functionality, or the joy of instant results, both the crock pot and oven methods offer robust solutions. They allow you to enjoy all the sensory experiences of soapmaking without the long wait times of traditional methods. The texture, the scent, and the immediate satisfaction of a usable product in just days can be incredibly motivating and inspiring. Embrace these techniques as you continue to explore and expand your soapmaking journey.

Finishing Touches for Hot Process Soaps

Finishing and the hot process transform a basic soap bar into a true work of art. When you've poured your hot process soap into the mold and it's had time to cool, it might not look like much. But with a bit of care, creativity, and some finishing techniques, your soap will be ready to impress family, friends, or even potential customers.

Let's start with the most basic step, which is *smoothing the top*. While the rustic, textured tops of hot process soaps have their charm, a smooth finish can give a more professional look. To achieve this, as soon as you've poured your soap into the mold, you can use a spatula to even out the surface. If you're aiming for a textured top, manipulate the surface with the spatula or a spoon to create peaks and valleys.

Once your soap has fully set, typically after 12 to 24 hours, it's time for *unmolding* and *cutting*. For the cleanest cuts, ensure your soap is completely cooled. Use a sharp knife or a soap cutter to slice your soap into bars. If you're selling or gifting these, you might want to measure each bar to ensure consistency in size and weight, which adds a professional touch.

Don't underestimate the power of *beveled edges*. By running a vegetable peeler along the edges of each bar, you can remove sharp corners, giving your soap a smoother, more polished appearance. Not only does this improve the look, but it also enhances the user experience, making the soap more comfortable to hold and use.

Adding *embellishments* to your soap can really set it apart. Consider pressing dried herbs, flowers, or botanicals on top of your soap while it's still soft enough to adhere. Just think about how lovely a lavender soap looks with sprigs of dried lavender on top, or a rose soap with delicate petals sprinkled across the surface. Make sure to choose botanicals that complement the essential oils and herbs used in your soap to create a cohesive aesthetic and aromatic experience.

If you're feeling more adventurous, you might try *stamping* your soap. You can use rubber stamps, but for a more durable option, consider investing in a soap stamp made specifically for this purpose. Stamping is best done when the soap has firmed up but is still slightly malleable. Lightly press the stamp into the soap's surface, and you'll find yourself with bars that carry your personal touch or even your brand's logo.

Buffing and polishing can add an extra level of finesse. After cutting your soap, let it cure for a few days to firm up. Then, using a soft cloth, gently buff each bar to a subtle shine. This extra step can

Essential Soaps

make your soaps look professionally finished and can be particularly appealing when presenting your soaps for sale.

Fragrance is often what people remember the most about a soap. That's why *adding finishing fragrances* is another essential touch. While you've already added essential oils during the soapmaking process, you can spritz a light mist of diluted essential oil on the bars just before they finish curing. This will ensure a lasting scent that will delight anyone who uses your soap.

Don't forget the finishing touch hidden within the soap: *superfatting*. This involves adding an extra amount of oils that don't fully saponify, resulting in a richer, more moisturizing bar. Your choice of superfatting oils—whether it's shea butter, almond oil, or coconut oil—can add unique benefits and enhance the luxurious feel of your soaps. See Chapter 8 for deeper insights into superfatting techniques.

Once your soap bars are cut, cured, and beautified, you might consider adding something that will last long after the soap itself is used up—*personal touches or branding elements*. Consider designing a logo or brand name that you can either stamp onto the soap or include on the packaging. You could also imbue your packaging with little extras like a handwritten note or special wrapping paper that matches the soap's scent or theme, discussed in more detail in Chapter 18.

Finalizing your hot process soaps isn't just about looks; it's also about practicality. Allow sufficient time for *curing*, even if hot process soaps don't require as long a cure time as cold process soaps. Giving your soap at least a week or two to fully harden will enhance its durability and longevity, ensuring a pleasant experience for the user.

Lastly, an important yet often overlooked step is the *quality check*. Before considering your batch complete, use a pH strip to test the soap to ensure it's skin-safe. A soap with a pH between 7 and 10 is safe and non-irritating. If the pH is too high, your soap may need a longer cure time or even to be rebatched to adjust the levels.

Finishing touches aren't just about appearance; they're part of crafting a luxurious, high-quality soap that stands out. Whether adding botanical embellishments, ensuring smooth edges, or buffing a shine, each finishing touch adds value and appeal, aligning with sustainable and eco-friendly practices that many soapmakers and users hold dear. Your final product is more than just soap; it's a handmade treasure reflective of your time, effort, and love for the craft.

Chapter 8: Superfatting and Saponification Explained

In this chapter, we'll delve into the intricacies of superfatting and saponification, pivotal concepts in the heart of soapmaking. Superfatting refers to adding extra fats or oils to your soap mixture beyond the amount needed for saponification, enriching your soap with nourishing properties that are gentle on the skin. This process not only enhances the moisturizing and emollient qualities of natural soap but also introduces an element of luxurious indulgence. Saponification, the chemical reaction that transforms fats and lye into soap, is crucial for ensuring your soap bars are both effective and safe. Understanding the balance between these two processes allows you to craft soaps that not only cleanse but also care for the skin, promoting a harmonious blend of efficacy and gentle luxury in every bar. Let's unlock the potential of superfatting and master the art of saponification to elevate your soapmaking skills and create products that truly stand out.

Saponification Values and Why They Matter

These are integral to understanding and perfecting your soapmaking craft. Whether you're a seasoned soapmaker or just starting, the concept of saponification values is essential knowledge that will elevate your soap creations. At its core, saponification is the chemical reaction that occurs when fats or oils come into contact with lye (sodium hydroxide), producing glycerol and soap. It's a process that's been used for centuries and is the fundamental backbone of all soapmaking.

The saponification value (SV) refers to the amount of lye required to completely saponify a given quantity of fat or oil. In essence, it's a measure of the fatty acid's reaction with a strong base to produce soap. Each type of oil or fat has a unique saponification value, which indicates the precise amount of lye needed to transform that oil into soap. Knowing these values is crucial not only for achieving the correct balance between lye and oils but also for ensuring the quality and safety of your final product. Soap that has too much lye can be harsh and irritating, while soap with too little lye can be too soft or oily.

Understanding saponification values allows you to customize your soap recipes with precision. For instance, olive oil has a saponification value of approximately 0.134, meaning that to saponify one gram of olive oil, you need about 0.134 grams of lye. On the other hand, coconut oil, known for its luxurious lather and cleansing properties, has a saponification value of around 0.183. By knowing these values, you can accurately calculate the lye necessary for different oils in your recipes, ensuring that your soap batch will solidify correctly and produce the desired texture and qualities.

When formulating your soap recipes, you'll often use a soap calculator to help determine the correct amount of lye based on the oils you select. These calculators are invaluable tools, allowing you to input the weight of each oil in your recipe and receive an accurate measurement of the required lye. This ensures that your soap will not only turn out as expected but will also be safe to use. Remember, safety is paramount when working with lye, and precise calculations are a key component in maintaining that safety.

In addition to safety and precision, understanding saponification values can also assist in achieving the desired properties in your soap. Different oils contribute different qualities:

hardness, cleansing ability, lathering, and moisturizing properties. Coconut oil, for example, produces a hard bar with a lot of lather, while olive oil results in a softer, more moisturizing bar. By knowing the saponification values of each oil, you can balance your recipes to combine these properties, creating a bespoke soap that meets your specific needs.

Moreover, understanding the saponification value is particularly important when working with a mix of oils. When creating a multi-oil soap recipe, each oil's saponification value must be considered to calculate the total lye amount accurately. For example, if your recipe includes olive oil, coconut oil, and shea butter, you'll need to calculate the lye for each oil separately and then sum these amounts to find the total lye required. This meticulous process ensures that each oil is fully saponified, resulting in a balanced and well-crafted soap.

In addition to these practical applications, grasping the concept of saponification values deepens your appreciation for the chemistry behind soapmaking. It's a fascinating process where intricate chemical reactions transform humble ingredients into a functional and luxurious product. This understanding can inspire creativity, allowing you to experiment with new oil combinations and further expand your soapmaking repertoire.

Let's not forget the role of sustainable and eco-friendly practices in modern soapmaking. Knowing your saponification values can help you make informed choices about the oils you use, potentially opting for more sustainable options. For example, while palm oil has a great balance of properties for soapmaking, it's widely known for its environmental impact. By understanding the saponification values of alternative oils, you can create palm-free recipes that are both effective and more environmentally responsible. This aligns perfectly with the growing movement towards sustainability and eco-conscious living, which many soapmakers are passionate about.

Furthermore, a firm grasp of saponification values enables the creation of unique soap formulations tailored to different skin types or preferences. For those with sensitive skin, you might choose oils with lower cleansing values and higher moisturizing properties. On the other hand, if you're crafting soap for oily skin, you might select oils known for their higher cleansing abilities. The knowledge of saponification values ensures you can tweak your recipes to cater to any specific skin needs.

Saponification values are also invaluable when scaling up your soapmaking efforts, whether you're producing for a small business or gifting larger quantities. Accurate calculations are essential to maintaining consistency across larger batches. Scaling up doesn't just mean using larger quantities of ingredients; it also means ensuring that your measures and ratios remain precise, so every bar of soap meets your established standards.

Consider this: the difference between a successful soap batch and a failure can come down to understanding and correctly applying saponification values. If the lye ratio is off, the soap could end up too caustic or too greasy. Mastering these calculations allows you to troubleshoot and refine your processes, ultimately leading to better products and a more enjoyable soapmaking experience. This knowledge empowers you to take control of every aspect of your soapmaking, from initial formulation to the final product.

In conclusion, saponification values are the bedrock of successful soapmaking. They are not just numbers but the keys to unlocking the full potential of your ingredients and creativity. By understanding and applying these values, you gain greater control over your recipes, ensure the safety and effectiveness of your soaps, and can experiment with new and innovative formulations. Embrace this knowledge, let it inform your creations, and enjoy the satisfaction of producing high-quality natural soaps that are as beneficial for your skin as they are for the environment.

Benefits of Superfatting Your Soap

Superfatting Your Soap can truly transform your soapmaking experience, elevating both the quality and luxurious feel of your final product. But before diving into the benefits, let's understand what superfatting is. Superfatting is the process of adding extra oils or fats to your soap formula beyond what's needed to completely saponify the lye. This method not only ensures a gentler, more moisturizing bar but also brings several other advantages that seasoned soapmakers and beginners alike will appreciate.

One of the most compelling benefits of superfatting is the increased moisturizing properties it imparts to the soap. When making soap, some of the lye is left unsaponified due to the extra fats, which means that these fats remain in the final bar. This creates a soap that's much kinder to the skin, leaving it softer and more hydrated. This can be particularly beneficial for those with dry or sensitive skin, as the extra oils can help to soothe and nourish.

Another significant advantage is the luxurious feel that superfatted soaps provide. The additional oils not only moisturize but also contribute to a richer, creamier lather. This can make the simple act of washing your hands or taking a shower feel like a pampering experience. For those making soap as gifts or for sale, this added luxury can be a unique selling point that sets your products apart from others on the market.

Superfatting also offers an opportunity to experiment and customize your soap recipes even further. Different oils and butters bring their distinct properties to the soap. For instance, adding shea butter can provide extra creaminess and conditioning properties, while a touch of cocoa butter can lend the bar a firmer texture and subtle chocolatey aroma. The endless possibilities for customization mean you can tailor your soaps to meet specific needs or preferences, whether you're aiming for anti-aging properties, deep moisturization, or even a specific scent profile.

However, it's not just about the luxurious feel and moisturizing benefits. Superfatting your soap can also enhance its healing properties. Ingredients like olive oil, avocado oil, and hemp seed oil are packed with vitamins, antioxidants, and essential fatty acids that can contribute to skin health. These oils can help create a soap that not only cleanses but also nurtures and repairs the skin, making it ideal for therapeutic and medicinal soaps aimed at treating skin conditions.

For artisanal soapmakers, superfatting can be a game-changer in terms of creativity. The technique allows for the incorporation of delicate, unsaponifiable oils that might otherwise be broken down by the lye. This opens up new avenues for using exotic oils and butters that bring their intrinsic properties and luxurious textures to the final product. It encourages experimentation with lesser-known but highly beneficial ingredients such as tamanu oil, meadowfoam seed oil, or murumuru butter.

In addition, superfatted soaps often have a better shelf life. The presence of unsaponified oils can act as a natural preservative, extending the longevity of the bar. This is particularly advantageous for small business owners who sell their soaps, as it ensures that the products remain fresh and effective for the end-users. It also offers peace of mind for individual soapmakers who don't want their carefully crafted bars to go to waste.

Superfatting also contributes to the overall sensory experience of using handmade soap. The added oils can introduce subtle scents and textures that aren't achievable with a fully-saponified formula. The gentle glide, the soft lather, the occasional whiff of a natural aroma—

all these elements work together to make the experience of using your soap something to look forward to every day.

It's important to note, however, that superfatting does require some additional calculation and precision. An improper balance of lye and oils can result in a bar that's either too harsh because of excess lye or too greasy due to uncombined oils. For those new to soapmaking, it may be beneficial to start with tested recipes that include superfatting as a standard part of the formula. Once comfortable, you can begin to experiment with your own custom recipes to see what superfatting levels produce your ideal bar of soap.

Moreover, superfatting your soap aligns perfectly with eco-friendly and sustainable practices. By focusing on natural oils and butters, you avoid synthetic chemicals and additives, making your soaps kinder to the environment as well as to your skin. This approach resonates with the growing consumer demand for sustainable and natural products and is a great way to contribute positively to the wellness and ecological movement.

In conclusion, the **benefits of superfatting your soap** are manifold. From creating a more moisturizing and luxurious bar to allowing for greater customization and experimentation, the advantages are substantial. Whether you're crafting soap for personal use or producing it commercially, superfatting can elevate your creations to new levels of quality and efficacy. So, embrace this technique, experiment with a variety of oils, and discover the alchemy that transforms simple ingredients into a bar of soap that's as beneficial for the skin as it is a joy to use.

Chapter 9: Essential Oils and Aromatherapy in Soapmaking

Introducing essential oils into your soapmaking process elevates your creations by blending therapeutic benefits with delightful fragrances. Essential oils, extracted from plants with potent properties, contribute not only to the scent but also offer a range of aromatherapy advantages. They can energize, soothe, or even aid in relaxation, depending on the oils chosen. For the soapmaker, mastery of essential oil blending is both an art and a science, requiring a keen understanding of each oil's unique profile. Always remember, safety is paramount—essential oils are powerful and must be used with respect to recommended dilutions and precautions to avoid adverse reactions. Harnessing these natural gifts, you will craft soaps that evoke a sensory experience, transforming everyday routines into a moment of indulgence and self-care. Ready to infuse your soap with the essence of nature? Let's dive in!

Essential Oil Safety and Usage

Safety around oils and their usage is crucial for anyone delving into the world of natural soapmaking. Essential oils are concentrated plant extracts that capture the natural fragrance and therapeutic properties of their source. While they can elevate your soap into a luxurious and aromatic experience, it's vital to handle them responsibly to ensure safety and efficacy.

Essential Soaps

One of the first considerations when using essential oils is understanding their potency. These oils are highly concentrated, often requiring just a few drops to impart their benefits. Overuse can result in soap that's not only overpowering in scent but also potentially irritating to the skin. A general rule of thumb is to use a dilution rate of 1-3% essential oil to the total weight of your soap base. For instance, in a 1-pound batch of soap, you'd use anywhere from 5 to 15 grams of essential oil.

Proper storage also plays a role in essential oil safety. Store your oils in dark glass bottles in a cool, dry place away from direct sunlight. This helps maintain their potency and extends shelf life. Exposure to heat, light, and air can degrade essential oils, altering their scent and efficacy. Always make sure to tightly seal the bottles after use to prevent oxidation and contamination.

When integrating essential oils into your soapmaking, it's also essential to be aware of each oil's flashpoint. The flashpoint is the temperature at which the oil can ignite. In soapmaking, particularly hot process methods, reaching a flashpoint can result in the evaporation of the essential oil or, worse, a fire hazard. Knowledge of flashpoints ensures that you add the oils at a safe stage of the process.

Allergies and sensitivities are another critical consideration. Some essential oils can cause allergic reactions or sensitivities, even in small amounts. Conduct a patch test before using a new essential oil in your soap. Apply a small diluted amount to a patch of skin and wait 24 hours to check for any reactions. This step is especially important if you plan to sell your soaps or gift them to others, as you want to ensure your products are safe for all users.

Some essential oils are also not recommended for use by certain populations, such as pregnant women, nursing mothers, infants, or those with specific health conditions. For instance, oils like peppermint, rosemary, and eucalyptus should be used with caution in these groups. If you fall into these categories or have customers who do, it's advisable to consult with a healthcare professional before using certain oils.

Moreover, not all essential oils are created equal. Quality can vary significantly between different brands and suppliers. Always source your oils from reputable suppliers who provide information about the oil's extraction method, country of origin, and purity. Look for therapeutic-grade oils and avoid those with synthetic additives or adulterants. This guarantees you're using oils that are true to their botanical origin and free of harmful substances.

A critical but often overlooked aspect of essential oil usage in soap is regulatory compliance. Depending on where you live, there may be guidelines and restrictions on the use of certain essential oils in cosmetics. In the United States, for instance, the Food and Drug Administration (FDA) has regulations on the labeling and use of essential oils. Always stay informed on the legal requirements in your area to ensure your products are both safe and compliant.

Blending essential oils can be an art form, but it also requires a good understanding of oil interactions. Some oils complement each other beautifully, creating complex and appealing fragrances. Others, however, may clash or produce an undesirable scent when combined. Begin with small test batches when experimenting with new blends to avoid wasting materials and ensure a harmonious final product.

Safety also extends to proper labeling and user instructions. Particularly if you're selling your soaps, clear labeling can inform your customers about the essential oils used in the product. Include any relevant safety information, such as potential allergens or usage precautions, to foster trust and transparency with your buyers.

In the end, essential oil safety and usage is about mindfulness and respect for these powerful extracts. With proper handling, storage, and usage, essential oils can significantly enrich your soapmaking endeavors, creating delightful and therapeutic products that both you and your customers will love. Always prioritize safety, educate yourself continuously, and enjoy the aromatic journey.

Blending Essential Oils for Fragrance

This involves the captivating art of aroma combination that transcends mere scent to evoke emotions and create experiences. Creating the perfect blend of essential oils ensures your soap not only cleanses but also delights the senses, giving each bar a unique personality. Let's journey through the enchanting world of essential oils and explore how to blend them harmoniously for fragrant, exquisite soaps.

To begin with, understanding the basics of essential oils is crucial. Essential oils are extracted from various parts of plants, such as flowers, leaves, and stems, capturing the plant's aromatic essence. Each oil has its distinct profile, consisting of top, middle, and base notes. These notes form the structure of your fragrance. Top notes are the first impression—light and refreshing. Middle notes, or "heart notes," emerge as the top notes fade, adding depth and fullness. Base notes linger the longest, providing a foundation that anchors the blend.

When crafting a fragrance blend, think of it as composing a symphony. Each oil plays its part harmoniously. Start by selecting a primary scent—this is typically your middle note. Complement this with top and base notes that enhance the primary aroma without overshadowing it. For example, consider blending lavender (middle note) with uplifting bergamot (top note) and grounding patchouli (base note). This trio creates a balanced, multi-layered fragrance.

Creating balanced blends requires patience and experimentation. It's often helpful to start with a small test batch. Use droppers to measure the oils in exact proportions—3 parts middle note, 2 parts top note, and 1 part base note is a common starting point. Remember, essential oils can vary in intensity, so a drop or two can significantly alter your blend. Document your experiments diligently to replicate successful blends later.

Another key element in blending essential oils is synergy. Some oils may enhance each other's properties when combined. For instance, blending eucalyptus and peppermint creates a refreshing and invigorating scent that's also notably beneficial for respiratory support. Synergy not only amplifies the fragrance but can also enhance the therapeutic benefits of your soap.

In addition to balance and synergy, you must consider the seasonality of your fragrances. Winter scents might include warming spices like cinnamon and clove, paired with sweet orange for a festive feel. Meanwhile, summer soaps could highlight cooling, fresh scents such as peppermint and lemon. Adjusting your blends according to the season allows you to offer a dynamic range of soaps that resonate with your customers' needs throughout the year.

Essential oil blending also opens up creative avenues. Don't hesitate to venture into uncharted territories with unique combinations. Perhaps you could mix a citrusy yuzu with spicy ginger and a hint of cedarwood for an exotic, invigorating soap. Monitor customer feedback and make iterative adjustments to refine your signature blends. Thus, you'll not only hone your craft but also build a loyal customer base who anticipates your new creations eagerly.

Safety should never be an afterthought when dealing with essential oils. Some oils, like citrus oils, can be photosensitive, making the skin more prone to sunburn. Others, such as cinnamon or clove, are potent and can cause skin irritation if not properly diluted. A general rule of thumb is to keep the total essential oil concentration in your soap to around 1-2% of the total weight of your soap batch to ensure safety and efficacy.

Essential Soaps

Additionally, always cross-reference your essential oils with credible sources to verify safe usage levels. Essential oils like tea tree, although widely benefits-laden, should be used judiciously. Pregnant women and individuals with specific health conditions should exercise caution and seek advice before using certain oils. Blending essential oils isn't just about achieving the perfect scent; it's about doing so responsibly.

Once you've formulated your blends, proper integration into your soap batch is the final key step. For cold process soaps, add essential oils at trace, the point when your soap mixture begins to thicken. In hot process soapmaking, add them after the cook when the soap has cooled slightly, preserving the integrity of the fragrance. Stir thoroughly to ensure even distribution throughout the soap.

Making fragrant soap is an immersive, rewarding process. Blending essential oils not only offers you creative freedom but also connects you closer to the natural world. Each time you infuse your soap with a custom fragrance, you're embedding a piece of your artistry and personality into every bar. And that, dear reader, is where the true magic of soapmaking lies.

With the right blend, you can transport the user to a blooming lavender field, a serene forest, or a beachfront paradise. So explore, experiment, and embrace the wonderful world of essential oils. Through your blends, you'll create soaps that are uniquely yours and immensely cherished by those who experience them.

Chapter 10:
Herbal Additives and Botanicals

Integrating herbal additives and botanicals into your soap recipes can transform a simple cleansing bar into a luxurious, spa-like experience. When you add herbs and botanicals, not only are you enhancing the visual appeal of your soaps, but you're also imparting a variety of skin-loving benefits and aromatic qualities. Whether you're infusing oils with the soothing properties of lavender, incorporating the anti-inflammatory benefits of calendula, or simply decorating the tops of your bars with dried rose petals, these natural elements can elevate your soapmaking to new heights. Selecting and using the right herbs, flowers, and plant materials involves understanding their unique properties and how they interact with your soap base. As you begin to experiment, you'll discover the endless possibilities these natural ingredients offer, transforming each batch into a work of art that nourishes the skin and delights the senses.

Infusing Oils With Herbs

Infusion is not just about adding fragrance and color to your soaps; it's about imbuing your products with the natural benefits and healing properties of herbs. This technique can transform your soapmaking practice, allowing you to create truly nourishing and therapeutic soaps. The process of infusing oils with herbs, while seemingly simple, holds the potential for endless creativity and customization. Whether you're a seasoned soapmaker or a budding enthusiast, infusing oils is a valuable skill in your soapmaking toolkit.

To begin with, you need to select your herbs wisely. The choice of herb depends on the properties you want to transfer to the oil and ultimately to your soap. For instance, if you desire a calming effect, lavender and chamomile are excellent choices. For their antibacterial properties, you might lean towards thyme or rosemary. Whatever herb you choose, ensure it is fully dried to prevent mold and bacteria growth during the infusion process.

The method of infusion can be as individual as the soapmaker themselves, with variables such as time, temperature, and technique affecting the end result. The cold infusion method is one of the most straightforward ways to infuse herbs into oils. Simply fill a glass jar about one-third full with dried herbs and then top it up with your choice of oil, leaving some space at the top of the jar. Olive oil is a popular base because of its widespread availability and beneficial properties, but other oils like coconut, almond, or jojoba also work well.

After sealing the jar tightly, store it in a cool, dark place for four to six weeks, shaking it gently every few days to help the infusion process. This slow method extracts the fullest flavor and medicinal properties from the herbs. Once the time has passed, strain the herbs from the oil using a fine mesh strainer or cheesecloth, ensuring you squeeze out every last drop of your precious infusion. The resulting infused oil can then be used as an ingredient in your soap recipes to add additional benefits and a gentle hue.

For those who may be short on time, the heat infusion method offers a faster alternative. In this method, combine your dried herbs and oil in a double boiler or a slow cooker set to a low temperature. Heat gently for two to three hours, monitoring closely to ensure the oil doesn't get too hot and the herbs don't burn. This method offers a quicker turnaround, though some argue it might compromise the quality of the infusion. Once the infusion is complete, strain the herbs out, and your oil is ready to use.

Temperature control is critical to the success of the heat infusion method. Oils should be kept at a relatively low heat – about 120°F to 140°F – to avoid degrading the beneficial properties of both the oil and the herbs. If you don't have a slow cooker with a temperature gauge, a double boiler on the stove can be a suitable alternative, provided you keep a close eye on the temperature. The key is a gentle and even heat throughout the infusion process.

Beyond these basic methods, you can experiment with other techniques like solar infusion, where you harness the power of the sun to gently warm your oil and herbs over several weeks. Simply place your jar of herbs and oil on a sunny windowsill and let nature do the work. This method requires patience and a bit of space, but the results can be incredibly rewarding, with a deep, rich infusion that reflects the slow but potent energy of the sun.

One of the beauties of infusing oils with herbs is the creative possibilities it opens up. You can combine different herbs to create custom blends tailored to specific skin types or needs. For instance, a blend of calendula, comfrey, and plantain creates a soothing oil perfect for sensitive or irritated skin. On the other hand, a mix of peppermint, eucalyptus, and tea tree can yield a refreshing, invigorating oil ideal for soaps meant to wake you up in the morning.

When it comes to selecting your base oils, the world is your oyster. Olive oil is a staple for its versatility and skin-loving properties, but don't hesitate to explore other oils like jojoba, which closely mimics the skin's natural sebum, or avocado oil, rich in vitamins and fatty acids. Each oil brings its own qualities to the final soap, and combining different oils can enhance those properties even further. For example, a combination of coconut oil and olive oil can create a balanced product with excellent moisturizing and cleansing properties.

Documentation is vital. Keep a detailed log of your infusing process, noting the herbs used, the type and amount of oil, infusion method, duration, and any observations about the final product. This helps in refining techniques and replicating successful batches. Photos can also provide a visual reference to see how the color and texture of the oil change over time, offering clues about the infusion's progress. Just as a chef keeps a recipe book, your infusing log becomes a valuable reference for creating consistent, high-quality soaps.

Infusing oils with herbs isn't just a practical technique; it's a bridge connecting you with traditions passed down through generations. Many cultures have utilized natural infusions for medicine and skincare for ages. By integrating these methods into your soapmaking, you're continuing a legacy that honors nature's wisdom. This connection to the past enriches the creative and therapeutic experience of making soap, contributing to the sustainability and mindfulness echoed throughout this book.

Furthermore, the environmental benefits are compelling. By choosing to infuse oils with herbs, you're reducing dependency on synthetic additives and fragrances. This not only benefits the skin but also promotes a healthier ecosystem by minimizing the chemical footprint of our creations. Infusing oils brings you closer to nature and reinforces the principles of eco-friendly and sustainable practices.

In conclusion, **Infusing Oils With Herbs** offers a world of opportunity for those passionate about soapmaking. Whether you're creating soaps for personal use or for a business, the ability to infuse oils with herbs enhances the quality, appeal, and efficacy of your products. It's a meticulous process that requires patience and attention to detail, but the results speak for themselves. Your soaps will not only cleanse the body but also nurture the soul, bringing a touch of nature's healing power into every bar.

Take time to experiment, explore different herbs and oils, and find combinations that resonate with you. Document your process, celebrate your successes, and learn from your experiments. The journey of infusing oils with herbs is one of continual learning and discovery, a journey that deepens your connection to the craft of soapmaking and the natural world. Happy infusing!

Selecting and Using Dried Herbs and Flowers

Dried Herbs and Flowers add not just beauty, but also therapeutic properties and delightful scents to your handcrafted soaps. Selecting the right herbs and flowers can elevate a basic bar of soap into a truly luxurious experience. But with so many options available, how do you choose? And how do you use them effectively in your soapmaking process? Let's explore the answers to these questions.

The key to selecting dried herbs and flowers lies in understanding their individual properties and how they interact with the soapmaking process. For instance, some herbs and flowers are known for their skin-soothing qualities, like calendula and chamomile, making them excellent choices for sensitive skin formulas. Others, such as rosemary and lavender, offer natural antibacterial and antifungal properties, which are ideal for facial soaps or foot scrubs.

Quality matters when selecting dried herbs and flowers. Always choose organic and sustainably sourced products whenever possible. Non-organic options can contain pesticides or other chemicals that may not only alter the appearance and scent of your soap but could also be harmful to the skin. Check with suppliers for certification or reliable sourcing if you're unsure.

When you start working with dried herbs and flowers, think about the aesthetic appeal they bring to your soap. Whole flower petals or small buds are visually striking, especially when set against a creamy bar of soap. On the other hand, finely ground herbs can add unique textures and subtle speckles throughout the soap. The choice between whole and ground forms often comes down to the final look and feel you're aiming for.

It's not just about looks, though. The way you incorporate dried herbs and flowers into your soap recipe can influence the overall product. Add too many, and you might end up with a crumbly bar or one that's scratchy on the skin. A good rule of thumb is to start with a small amount and adjust based on your results. Generally, 1 to 2 teaspoons of dried herbs or flowers per pound of soap base is a good starting point.

How you prepare your herbs and flowers for soapmaking also matters. Some dried herbs and flowers can brown or lose their color if added directly to the soap. To prevent this, infuse the herbs in your chosen oils before adding them to the lye solution. This not only helps retain the color but can also infuse your soap with deeper, more resilient scents. Infusing oils can be done by placing your dried botanicals in a jar, covering them with oil, and letting them steep for several weeks, then straining out the solids before use.

Another technique is adding dried herbs and flowers at trace—when your soap mixture has thickened to the consistency of pudding. At this stage, you can gently fold in the botanicals, ensuring even distribution throughout the batter. This method works particularly well for delicate herbs that might not withstand the high temperatures of the saponification process.

If you're incorporating flowers like rose petals or lavender buds, a helpful tip is to crush them slightly before adding them to your soap mixture. This can prevent them from floating to the top of your soap molds, ensuring they are evenly distributed in the final bar. Using a mortar and pestle or even your hands will do the trick.

Besides aesthetics and therapeutic properties, consider the aroma potential of your dried herbs and flowers. While essential oils will carry the bulk of the fragrance, the subtle scents of dried botanicals can complement and enhance these predominant notes. For example, combining dried lavender with lavender essential oil can intensify the calming aroma, making the soap experience even more soothing.

Seasonal variations also offer unique opportunities. Think about using dried citrus peels and calendula in your summer soaps for a fresh, sunny vibe or going for warming herbs like cinnamon and clove in your winter formulations. This not only makes your soap more appealing but can also help in marketing seasonal lines if you're selling your creations.

Experimenting with dried herbs and flowers opens the door to endless creativity. Document your experiments meticulously, noting the types and quantities of botanicals used, their effects on the texture and appearance of the soap, and, of course, the feedback from those who use your soap. This will build a wealth of knowledge that you can draw upon for future projects.

Sourcing your dried herbs and flowers can be another exciting part of the process. Many soapmakers cultivate their own botanicals, ensuring a fresh and organic supply. A small herb garden or even a few potted plants can yield a surprising amount of material over time. Harvest your herbs at their peak—usually just before they flower—for the most potent properties. After harvesting, dry them by hanging bundles in a cool, dark place or using a dehydrator for faster results.

While growing your own herbs is rewarding, there's also a community aspect to consider. Local farmers' markets, herbalists, and co-ops can be excellent sources for high-quality dried herbs and flowers. Engaging with these communities not only supports local businesses but also opens doors to collaboration and education.

In summary, **Selecting and Using Dried Herbs and Flowers** in your soapmaking is a delightful blend of artistry and science. It requires a keen eye for quality, an understanding of how different botanicals behave in soap, and a willingness to experiment and innovate. Whether you're incorporating chamomile for its calming properties, adding visual flair with rose petals, or infusing oils with rosemary for an invigorating scent, the possibilities are as vast as your imagination. Embrace the journey, keep learning, and let your creativity flourish as you transform simple soap into something truly extraordinary.

Chapter 11: Natural Colorants and Clays

Incorporating natural colorants and clays into your soap can elevate both its aesthetic appeal and its beneficial properties. Using clays like bentonite, kaolin, and French green not only provides stunning hues ranging from soft pastels to striking earth tones but also introduces skin-loving minerals that gently cleanse and exfoliate. Plant-based colorants offer a vibrant spectrum, from the golden warmth of turmeric to the deep magenta of madder root and the serene green of spirulina. These natural ingredients allow you to create soaps that are visually captivating while boasting the nourishing qualities your skin craves. Harnessing the power of nature's palette, you can craft unique bars that tell a story, whether you're striving for a calming lavender-infused creation or an invigorating peppermint and spirulina blend. By blending these elements thoughtfully, you're not just adding color, but also infusing each bar with a touch of nature's artistic and therapeutic essence.

Using Clays for Color and Texture

This is a revelation for any soapmaking enthusiast looking to take their creations to the next level. Not only do clays offer a natural way to add vibrant colors and intriguing textures to your soaps, but they also provide additional skincare benefits that synthetic additives can't match. Whether you're aiming for a rustic, earthy look or a refined, luxurious finish, the strategic use of clays can help you achieve that perfect aesthetic.

Clays come in a variety of types and colors, each with its own unique properties and benefits. Common options include kaolin (white clay), bentonite (gray or cream), French green clay, rose clay (pink), and Moroccan red clay. Each of these clays can impart a distinct hue to your soap, ranging from soft pastels to rich, deep tones. The color intensity will vary depending on the amount of clay used, allowing you to experiment and find the perfect balance for your designs.

The benefits of clays extend far beyond aesthetics. Kaolin clay, for instance, is known for its gentle cleansing properties and is particularly suitable for sensitive skin. Bentonite clay has excellent detoxifying abilities, making it ideal for oily or acne-prone skin types. French green clay is lauded for its ability to draw out impurities, while rose clay boasts a gentle touch that's perfect for mature or dry skin. Adding these clays to your soap doesn't just enhance appearance; it also boosts the skin-nourishing qualities of your final product.

When incorporating clays into your soap recipes, it's crucial to consider their absorbent nature. Clays can absorb liquid, which means they can slightly affect the texture and moisture content of your soap. To counteract this, mix your chosen clay with a small amount of water or oil before adding it to your soap batter. This pre-hydration step helps to evenly distribute the clay and minimizes the risk of clumping, ensuring a smooth and even finish.

Let's talk technique. In cold process soapmaking, you can add clay to the lye-water mixture or directly to the oils. Each method has its advantages. Adding clay to the lye-water may help in creating a more uniform color, especially for larger batches. On the other hand, adding it to the oils allows for more precise control over the final product's texture. Whichever method you choose, always sift the clay first to break up any lumps and ensure a consistent mix.

For melt and pour soapmaking, the process is a bit different. Because pre-made soap bases already have a set moisture content and consistency, it's best to adhere to a lower clay inclusion rate—roughly 1-3 teaspoons per pound of soap base. Melt the soap base gently, then add the pre-hydrated clay, stirring thoroughly to avoid any settling or clumping.

Layering and swirling techniques can further elevate your use of clays. Layering allows you to create distinct bands of color and texture within your soap, while swirling integrates multiple hues into intricate, marble-like patterns. To create a swirl effect, divide your soap batter into separate portions, mix each with a different type of clay, and then pour them together into your mold using a swirling motion. Utilize tools like skewers or chopsticks to draw additional patterns on the surface of your soap, allowing your clay colors to blend artfully.

Texture in soap is another avenue where clays truly shine. They offer a subtle, natural exfoliation that can enhance the sensory experience of using the soap. The fine, mineral-rich particles provide a gentle scrub, making your soap not just a cleansing agent but also a mild exfoliant. This dual functionality can be particularly appealing to customers looking for multi-benefit skincare products.

Safety and precision are key when working with clays. While they are generally safe to use, it's important to wear a mask when handling dry clay powders, as inhalation could irritate your respiratory system. Always ensure your workspace is well-ventilated and your tools are clean to avoid contamination. Accurate measurement is crucial too; too much clay can make your soap crumbly, while too little might not yield the desired coloring and benefits.

In essence, clays are a fantastic, multifunctional ingredient in the realm of natural soapmaking. They offer an eco-friendly, sustainable option for adding color and texture, without relying on synthetic materials. For small business owners, this can be a significant selling point, attracting customers who are mindful of the ingredients and sustainability of the products they purchase. Even for hobbyists, the experimentation with different clays can provide endless creative satisfaction.

Over time, you might find yourself leaning towards certain clays or combinations thereof, depending on the type of soap and its intended use. Don't hesitate to document your experiments and refine your techniques. The world of clays in soapmaking is vast and varied, and there's always something new to learn and explore.

Lastly, remember that soapmaking is not just a craft; it's a form of self-expression and a journey in sustainable living. Using clays for color and texture embodies these principles, allowing you to produce beautiful, functional soap bars while honoring the natural world. Whether you're creating soaps to use at home, to give as gifts, or to sell, the incorporation of clays can truly set your products apart, both in terms of aesthetics and skincare benefits.

Plant-Based Colorants: Roots, Berries, and Leaves

Colorants are some of the most exciting and versatile ingredients you can use in your soapmaking journey. Not only do they offer a wide array of vibrant colors that can transform your soaps into eye-catching works of art, but they also come with their own sets of beneficial properties. Using plant-based colorants aligns beautifully with the goal of creating all-natural, eco-friendly, and sustainable products. Let's dive into the world of natural dyes and explore how you can harness the coloring power of roots, berries, and leaves.

One of the simplest ways to start experimenting with plant-based colorants is by using roots. Turmeric root, for example, can impart a warm golden or light orange hue, depending on the amount used. Turmeric also comes with anti-inflammatory properties, making it a fantastic additive for soothing skin. To incorporate it, simply blend the powdered turmeric into your oil mixture or add it directly to your soap batter. Remember, a little goes a long way — too much can stain the skin or result in a rather overpowering scent.

Another wonderful root to consider is madder root, which has been used as a dye for centuries. Madder root powder can give your soaps a range of colors from soft pinks to deep reds. You can infuse your oils with madder root powder beforehand or add it directly into your soap mixture. For cold process soapmakers, adding the powder at trace can produce vibrant results. While experimenting with madder root, make sure to test small batches first to understand how it interacts with different oils and additives in your recipe.

In addition to roots, berries offer another palette of colors. Elderberries and blackberries, for example, can provide unique shades ranging from deep purples to blues. To use these berries, you can create a berry-infused water or oil, which you then incorporate into your soap recipe. Keep in mind that these types of colorants may fade over time, so consider using a higher concentration initially to ensure lasting color. The natural antioxidants in berries can also add a subtle level of skin-loving benefits to your soap.

If berry colors excite you, don't overlook the potential of purple or dark-colored grapes. Grape skin powder can be a useful coloring agent and is rich in antioxidants like resveratrol, giving an additional health benefit to your soap. Similar to other berries, use grape skin powder in moderation to achieve a lovely purple hue. Combine this ingredient with essential oils like lavender or chamomile to create soaps that are calming and nourishing.

Leaves are another excellent source of natural color. Stinging nettle powder, for instance, yields a vibrant green when added to soap. Not only does it bring a lovely color, but nettle is also believed to help with skin conditions such as eczema and acne. Spirulina, a type of blue-green algae, can also be used to achieve a rich green color. Spirulina is packed with nutrients and antioxidants, making it a superb addition to your natural soap recipes.

For more subtle, earthy tones, consider using spinach or parsley powder. These can produce soft greens that blend beautifully with natural soap bases. The chlorophyll in these leaves adds another layer of skin care benefits, providing soothing and anti-inflammatory effects. To achieve the best results, always make sure to strain any large particles from leaf infusions to avoid an unappealing texture in your soap.

Developing a keen understanding of these plant-based colorants will allow you to create a range of hues and designs. You can blend different powders, infusions, and extracts to achieve multi-toned soaps that are not only pleasing to the eye but beneficial to the skin. For instance, combining turmeric with a bit of spirulina can produce a beautiful, earthy green with golden swirls. Experimentation is key, and the best part is that the options are virtually endless.

For soapmakers who prefer more control over the final color, consider using natural micas that are tinted with plant-based dyes. These micas give you the ability to achieve consistent colors while still adhering to a natural approach. They can be especially helpful when you're looking to sell your soaps and need to maintain a certain level of product uniformity. Just be sure to check that the mica has been ethically sourced and naturally dyed.

On the practical side, keep in mind that natural colorants can behave differently depending on the soapmaking method you're using. Cold process soaps might show color variations due to the high pH level, which can cause some natural dyes to morph into unexpected shades. Hot process methods generally yield more stable and predictable results, making them ideal for those who want consistent color outcomes. Melt and pour bases are also an excellent choice for beginners interested in plant-based colorants, as they allow for greater control over the final look and feel of the soap.

Another tip is to bear in mind the natural scent that these colorants might bring to your soaps. While some, like turmeric and nettle, have a mild and earthy smell that blends well with various essential oils, others like berry powders can have a more noticeable aroma. Balancing these scents with complementary essential oils can enhance the overall experience of your soap, making it both visually and olfactorily appealing.

Incorporating plant-based colorants into your soapmaking repertoire offers endless possibilities for creativity and self-expression. By using roots, berries, and leaves, you're not only crafting beautiful soaps but also embracing a sustainable and eco-friendly practice that's kinder to our planet. Allow your imagination to run wild as you mix and match these natural ingredients to produce stunning, one-of-a-kind soaps that reflect your personal style and values.

Chapter 12: Exfoliants and Texturizers

Incorporating exfoliants and texturizers into your homemade soaps can elevate both their aesthetic and functional appeal, turning an ordinary bar into a luxurious experience. Whether you're looking to add a gentle scrub to your soap or seeking to craft an eye-catching texture, there are a plethora of natural options at your disposal. From finely ground oatmeal and delicate seeds to coarse sea salt and natural loofah, each ingredient brings its own unique properties and benefits. Selecting the right exfoliant or texturizer depends on the intended use of the soap and the skin type of its user. By thoughtfully integrating these elements, you can create soaps that not only cleanse but also invigorate the skin, offering a wholesome, spa-like feel right at home. Embrace the creativity and experimentation in blending various exfoliants to cater to different exfoliation needs—from light, everyday use to invigorating deep cleanses—ensuring each soap craft becomes a delightful sensory experience.

Choosing the Right Exfoliant

The right exfoliant is crucial for creating a soap that not only cleanses but also rejuvenates the skin. Exfoliants help slough away dead skin cells, promoting the regeneration of new cells and leaving the skin looking fresh and youthful. Whether you're aiming to add a gentle polish or a more vigorous scrub, the right exfoliant can be the key to achieving the desired texture and effectiveness in your bars of soap.

There's a vast array of exfoliants available, each serving different purposes and providing various benefits. If you're new to soapmaking, you might feel overwhelmed by the choices. However, understanding the properties of each type of exfoliant can make your decision easier. Broadly speaking, exfoliants fall into three categories: natural, synthetic, and mineral-based. For the purposes of natural, herb-infused soapmaking, we'll focus exclusively on natural exfoliants.

When considering *botanical exfoliants*, options such as ground oats, almond meal, and pumice might come to mind. Oats and almond meals are milder and suitable for sensitive skin, providing a gentle exfoliation that's perfect for everyday use. Ground pumice, on the other hand, offers a more thorough scrub due to its granular texture, making it ideal for soaps intended for tougher areas like feet.

Nutshell powders, like walnut or apricot kernel, provide a medium level of exfoliation. These are excellent for creating facial soaps or body bars meant to be used a couple of times a week. They help in gently removing dead skin cells without causing irritation or damage to the skin's surface.

Seeds and grains also make for excellent natural exfoliants. Poppy seeds, for instance, can add not only exfoliation but also a visual appeal to your soaps. Similarly, chia seeds and flax seeds can be used for their gentle scrubbing capabilities and aesthetic texture. Remember to consider the size and hardness of the seeds; softer seeds are better for facial soaps, while harder seeds can be more suited for body bars.

Let's not forget the benefits of using **herbal additives** as exfoliants. Dried and ground herbs like rosemary, lavender buds, and chamomile can provide a mild scrub while also imparting their beneficial properties to the soap. These herbs add both physical exfoliation and therapeutic benefits, making them an excellent dual-purpose ingredient.

Another popular category is **salt and sugar**, which can create robust, invigorating scrubs. Sea salt, Himalayan pink salt, and Epsom salts are great for making salt bars that can deeply cleanse and detoxify the skin. Sugar, especially brown sugar, offers a softer exfoliation and is often used in combination with oils and butters to create luxurious, exfoliating soap bars. However, it's essential to be mindful of humidity levels during storage to prevent salt and sugar from absorbing moisture and dissolving prematurely.

For a more eco-friendly option, consider using **coffee grounds**. Recycled coffee grounds provide a vigorous scrub and are known for their ability to help reduce the appearance of cellulite thanks to their caffeine content. Plus, there's the added benefit of repurposing a common household waste product, promoting a zero-waste lifestyle.

The choice of exfoliant often depends on the specific function and audience for your soap. If you are crafting soap for a luxurious, spa-like experience, you might opt for fine-ground botanicals and oatmeal, which provide gentle exfoliation suitable for most skin types. On the other hand, for a more utilitarian soap meant for gardeners or mechanics, coarser options like ground pumice or coffee grounds would be appropriate for heavy-duty scrubbing.

Incorporating the exfoliant into your soap recipe is straightforward but requires a bit of finesse to get the balance right. Too much exfoliant can make the soap gritty and uncomfortable to use, while too little might not provide the desired scrub. A general rule of thumb is to add about 1 tablespoon of exfoliant per pound of soap base, but this can vary based on the type of exfoliant and your personal preference. Remember, it's always easier to add more if needed rather than trying to compensate for an over-zealous pour.

The *timing* of adding your exfoliant to the soap mix also matters. For melt and pour soaps, you'll want to add the exfoliant just before pouring the soap into molds to ensure even distribution. For cold and hot process soaps, the exfoliant is typically added at trace or during the molding stage. Be sure to stir thoroughly to avoid clumping and ensure a consistent texture throughout each bar.

Testing and experimentation play a significant role in soapmaking. Don't hesitate to try different combinations and observe how they affect the final product. Different exfoliants interact uniquely with various oils, lye concentrations, and curing times. Keeping a detailed log of your experiments can help you refine your recipes and create the perfect balance for your signature soaps.

Finally, when choosing an exfoliant, consider any potential *allergies and sensitivities* your users might have. While many natural ingredients are gentle, some individuals may have allergic reactions to certain botanicals, nuts, or seeds. Being aware of this and offering clear labeling and ingredient lists can help you create products that are safe and enjoyable for a broader audience.

Choosing the right exfoliant brings with it an opportunity to craft custom soap that meets your exact needs or those of your clientele. Whether you're seeking to make a soothing facial bar, a vigorous scrub for hardworking hands, or a luxurious spa-like treat, there's an exfoliant that can help you achieve your goals. Let your creativity guide you, and don't be afraid to experiment and innovate. The world of natural exfoliants is vast and varied, offering endless possibilities for the dedicated soapmaker.

Incorporating Seeds, Salts, and Powders

Adding these to your soapmaking routine can elevate your artisan soaps to an entirely new level. These natural additives don't just enhance the aesthetic appeal of your bars; they add unique textures and provide various skin benefits that your customers are sure to love. When you carefully select and incorporate these ingredients, you transform a simple soap into a luxurious skincare product that promotes wellness and natural beauty.

The addition of seeds, salts, and powders offers a range of textures and exfoliating properties. Ingredients like poppy seeds, chia seeds, and cranberry seeds will gently scrub away dead skin cells, leaving the skin refreshed. These seeds are ideal for people looking for soaps with mild exfoliants. Remember, not all seeds are created equal. Poppy seeds, for instance, are tiny and smooth, making them great for everyday use, while larger seeds like cranberry offer a more robust exfoliation that's perfect for occasional use.

Himalayan pink salt and *sea salt* bring a different dimension to your soaps. These salts can help to draw toxins out from the skin and improve circulation. As salts dissolve, they provide a unique, spa-like experience that many users find beneficial. Incorporating salts into soap requires some care, as their granular nature can be abrasive if not mixed properly or measured correctly. Balance is key—too much salt can lead to a gritty texture that may be uncomfortable to use, while too little will diminish the soap's benefits. Also, remember to test the soap yourself or get feedback from others to fine-tune the ratio for optimal comfort and effectiveness.

Nourishing powders like oatmeal, almond, and charcoal are essential in creating soaps that cater to a variety of skin needs. Oatmeal powder is especially known for its soothing properties, perfect for sensitive skin types that are prone to irritation. It's fantastic for calming inflamed skin and providing gentle exfoliation. Almond powder, with its fine texture, adds a luxurious feel and is packed with vitamins that support skin health. Activated charcoal powder, on the other hand, is a powerful detoxifier known for drawing out impurities and toxins from the skin, making it a popular choice for facial soaps and soaps aimed at oily or acne-prone skin.

Integrating these additives into your soapmaking process is relatively straightforward but requires some attention to detail. Seeds are best added at trace, which is the point where the soap mixture has thickened sufficiently but is still pourable. Add them gradually, ensuring even distribution throughout the batch. Similarly, salts can be added at trace but take care to mix them well to avoid clumping or uneven distribution. With powders, it's often beneficial to blend them with a bit of your oils or liquids before incorporating them into the main mixture, ensuring they are well integrated and don't form lumps.

Here's a breakdown of some popular seeds, salts, and powders you might consider incorporating into your recipes:

- **Poppy Seeds:** Provide gentle exfoliation, great for face and body soaps.

- **Chia Seeds:** Known for their hydrating properties, they add a distinctive texture.

- **Himalayan Pink Salt:** Adds color and detoxifying benefits, ideal for creating "salt bars."

- **Oatmeal Powder:** Soothes and calms inflamed or sensitive skin.

- **Activated Charcoal:** Detoxifies skin; often used in facial and acne-prone skin soaps.

Incorporating these ingredients challenges you to experiment and find the perfect balance. For instance, a luxurious spa soap might combine Himalayan pink salt for detoxification, lavender seeds for gentle exfoliation, and oatmeal powder for soothing properties. Experimenting with combinations lets you discover unique and high-performing soap recipes.

Additionally, it's crucial to consider the appearance of your final product when adding seeds, salts, and powders. These elements can create beautiful visual effects as well as functional benefits. Take, for example, the interplay of white sea salt against the backdrop of deep charcoal soap. Such contrasts not only add aesthetic appeal but also make your soap stand out in a crowded marketplace. Carefully layering or swirling these ingredients can produce intricate designs that showcase your craftsmanship.

Another aspect to consider is how these additives affect your soap's shelf life. Salt has natural preservative qualities, helping to extend the lifespan of your soap bars. Powders like oatmeal, however, are more susceptible to moisture and should be stored in airtight containers until they're ready to be used.

Safety and sourcing are paramount. Always opt for high-quality, food-grade ingredients and be mindful of potential allergens. Some individuals may have sensitivities to certain seeds or botanical powders. Therefore, providing ingredient lists and sourcing information to your customers can enhance trust and transparency.

From the perspective of sustainable and eco-friendly practices, using natural exfoliants like seeds, salts, and powders eliminates the need for plastic microbeads, which are harmful to waterways and aquatic life. As crafters committed to sustainability, we can influence consumer choices by opting for ingredients that are safe for both skin and the environment.

In summary, incorporating seeds, salts, and powders into your soapmaking repertoire not only expands the variety and functionality of your products but also resonates with consumers seeking natural, effective, and environmentally responsible skincare solutions. Your creativity and attention to detail will result in soap bars that are not just cleansing tools but also sensory experiences that enhance everyday well-being.

Chapter 13:
Milk Soaps and Alternative Liquids

Milk soaps and alternative liquids provide a delightful twist to traditional soapmaking, offering unique benefits and textures that elevate the sensory experience of your creations. Integrating milks, like goat or coconut milk, into your soap not only enhances its creamy lather but also imparts nourishing properties that pamper the skin. Whether you're crafting soaps for personal use or for your small business, experimenting with teas, juices, and even beer can introduce intriguing textures and subtle hues, making your soap truly one-of-a-kind. Harnessing these uncommon liquids can transform your soap into a luxurious treat while promoting eco-friendly practices by utilizing local and sustainable ingredients. Embrace the endless possibilities, and let your creativity flow as you explore the art of milk soaps and alternative liquids.

Making Soap with Milk

Milk can add a luxurious, creamy texture to your homemade soaps, enriching them with nourishing qualities that are perfect for all skin types. Milk soaps are beloved for their moisturizing, gentle characteristics, making them highly sought after by those with sensitive or dry skin. Incorporating milk into your soap recipes isn't just about texture; it can also infuse your bars with vitamins, minerals, and proteins that aid in skin health.

Essential Soaps

The journey of incorporating milk into soap starts with selecting the right type of milk. There's a wide variety to choose from, each bringing its own unique benefits and properties. Goat milk, for instance, is a popular choice due to its high fat content, which increases the creaminess of the soap. It is also rich in vitamins A and D, essential for skin repair and rejuvenation. Cow milk, readily available and cost-effective, provides good hydration and contains lactic acid, which can help with gentle exfoliation.

Don't overlook plant-based milk alternatives like almond, coconut, or oat milk. These options cater to those looking for vegan formulas and also contribute valuable nutrients to the soap. Almond milk is known for its high vitamin E content, beneficial for skin elasticity and repair. Coconut milk brings a lush, foamy lather and an extra dose of moisturizing properties, while oat milk is incredibly soothing, ideal for inflamed or irritated skin.

One of the challenges of using milk in soapmaking is managing temperature control. Milk can scorch when exposed to high heat, leading to discoloration and an unpleasant burnt smell. The key is to freeze your milk before beginning the soapmaking process. By freezing the milk into ice cube-sized pieces, you keep the temperature down when you mix it with lye, thus preventing it from overheating.

Let's dive into the specifics of preparing a goat milk soap recipe. Start by measuring your milk and pouring it into ice cube trays. Once frozen, slowly combine these milk cubes with your lye, stirring gently. Although the reaction will generate heat, the solid state of the milk helps to keep the mixture cool and maintain its cream color.

After successfully creating your lye-milk mixture, it's time to add the oils. Combine your chosen oils and fats, heating them gently until they are fully melted and blended. Different oils bring different qualities to your soap; olive oil for conditioning, coconut oil for a good lather, and shea butter for an added moisture boost.

Once your oils are ready, carefully mix them with the lye-milk solution. At this stage, you can add essential oils and other additives to customize the soap's fragrance, color, and texture. Lavender essential oil pairs beautifully with goat milk, bringing a calming scent and additional therapeutic benefits. Other great combiantions include honey, which acts as a natural humectant, drawing moisture into the skin.

Achieving the perfect trace is crucial with milk soaps. Keep blending until the mixture thickens to the consistency of a light custard. Pour the mixture into molds and allow it to sit. The curing time for milk soaps can vary, but a general rule of thumb is to let it sit for four to six weeks to ensure it hardens completely and reaches the ideal pH level for skin usage.

During the curing process, observe the soap for any unusual spots or odors. If the milk had an unexpected response to the lye, you might see orange spots or experience a sour smell. These are indicators that the soap may have developed DOS (Dreaded Orange Spot) or has gone rancid. To minimize this, ensure your work environment is clean and that you're using fresh, high-quality ingredients.

Creating soap with milk can feel like a meticulous chemistry experiment, but the rewards are well worth it. The end product is gentle, luxurious, and full of beneficial nutrients for the skin. As you gain experience, you may want to experiment with combining different kinds of milk or adding ingredients like clays and exfoliants for an even richer bar.

Milk soaps offer endless possibilities for artistry and customization. For instance, camel milk and donkey milk have become exotic alternatives, each with its own set of skin-loving properties. These premium ingredients can make your soap stand out in a crowded market, offering a unique selling point for your soapmaking business.

Remember, practice and patience are key when working with milk in soapmaking. Each batch becomes a learning experience, helping you refine your process and achieve more consistent results. Embrace the creativity and the potential mistakes—each one brings you closer to mastering the art.

As you become more comfortable with milk soaps, don't shy away from exploring other alternative liquids like teas, juices, and herbal infusions. These can further enhance your soap with unique properties and benefits, complementing the nurturing qualities that milk brings to the table.

Incorporating milk into your soapmaking repertoire broadens your creative horizons and allows you to craft bars that cater to a diverse audience with different skin needs and preferences. Whether for personal use or as a product offering, milk soaps deliver a blend of luxury, nourishment, and artistry that's hard to beat.

Using Teas, Juices, and Other Liquids

Adding Teas, Juices, and Other Liquids in soapmaking isn't just a creative endeavor; it's a doorway to a world of possibilities. Imagine infusing your soaps with the calming properties of chamomile tea or the vibrant colors and antioxidants found in fresh vegetable juices. These natural liquids not only provide unique colors and fragrances but also bring a host of skin benefits that align perfectly with the ethos of eco-friendly and sustainable practices in DIY soapmaking.

Starting with teas, they're among the easiest to incorporate, offering an array of benefits depending on your choice. Herbal teas like mint, lavender, and chamomile can imbue your soap with soothing and relaxing properties. For a more invigorating experience, consider green tea or black tea, which bring antioxidants and a subtle, earthy aroma. To begin, simply brew a strong tea, strain out the leaves, and allow it to cool to room temperature before adding it to your soap recipe in place of water.

When using teas, you'll also notice a change in color, adding an extra layer of aesthetic appeal to your handmade soaps. For instance, chamomile tea adds a gentle yellow hue, while green tea leaves might give your soap a soft, natural green color. Furthermore, keeping the tea leaves intact can provide a natural, gentle exfoliation if included in the mix. Don't be afraid to experiment with combinations; a blend of different teas can create a multifaceted and unique bar of soap.

Moving on to juices, these offer a realm of vibrant possibilities. Freshly squeezed fruit and vegetable juices are packed with beneficial enzymes, vitamins, and minerals. Carrot juice, for instance, is rich in beta-carotene, providing a rich orange color and promoting healthy skin. Cucumber juice can be added for its soothing and hydrating properties, making it ideal for facial soaps. Remember, though, while juices add a fantastic array of benefits, they also contain sugars which can accelerate the saponification process, leading to a quicker trace.

It's essential to handle juices with care. Due to their high sugar content, juices can cause the soap to overheat if not properly managed. A helpful tip is to refrigerate or even partially freeze the juice before mixing it with lye. This way, the lower starting temperature can help control the heat during the chemical reaction. Additionally, be prepared to stir more frequently as the soap mixture may thicken faster than usual.

Other unique liquids like coconut water, aloe vera juice, and even beer and wine offer distinct advantages and require careful handling as well. Coconut water is hydrating and can create a rich lather in soaps, while aloe vera juice is known for its soothing and healing properties, perfect for sensitive skin formulations. When using these liquids, much like with juices, the sugar content needs to be considered. Using aloe vera gel, for example, might require you to adjust the amount of lye to ensure proper saponification.

For those looking to explore more creative avenues, adding beer or wine can be a fantastic option. Beer soap often features a rich, foamy lather and can add a depth of color and fragrance to the final product. Similarly, wine, especially red wine, can introduce antioxidants and a beautiful, deep color. The alcohol content in these beverages usually needs to be boiled off before being used in soapmaking to avoid a volatile reaction with lye. Once that's done, the remaining liquid can serve as a wonderful base for your soap.

Deciding which liquid to use boils down to what you want your soap to convey—both aesthetically and therapeutically. For example, a combination of aloe vera and green tea can create a soap that's both rejuvenating and nourishing. Or perhaps you're interested in a morning pick-me-up bar with coffee or espresso, taking advantage of caffeine's reputed skin-firming properties while enjoying the added exfoliation from coffee grounds.

As you experiment, keep meticulous notes on the proportions and outcomes. Different liquids can change the texture, set time, and even curing requirements of your soap. Balance is key; sometimes, combining a primary liquid with a bit of distilled water can provide the consistency and balance needed for a successful batch.

Let's not forget the impact these natural liquids have on the environment and sustainability efforts. By opting for teas, juices, and other natural liquids over synthetic ingredients, you're actively reducing your carbon footprint. Many of these ingredients can be sourced locally or made at home, ensuring that you're not only creating a high-quality product but also supporting a more sustainable way of living.

In conclusion, incorporating teas, juices, and other liquids into your soapmaking adds depth and character to your creations, unlocking benefits that go beyond mere aesthetics. Whether you're crafting for personal use or considering expanding into a small business, these natural options provide enhanced value for both your products and your customers. With careful preparation and a sense of adventure, you can create luxurious soaps that not only cleanse but also nourish and delight the senses.

Chapter 14:
Vegan and Palm-Free Soap Options

Venturing into vegan and palm-free soap options is a delightful way to blend ethical choices with creative soapmaking. Imagine crafting bars that nourish the skin while honoring the planet; it's simpler than you might think. Swapping traditional animal fats and palm oil for sustainable plant-based oils like olive, coconut, and shea butter opens up a world of possibilities, each contributing unique properties to your soap. With a little experimentation, you'll find combinations that create lather-rich, moisturizing soaps showcasing nature's bounty without compromising on your principles. The key is to understand the balance of hardness, cleansing properties, and conditioning power, selecting ingredients that reflect both your ethos and aesthetic goals. Choices such as using cocoa butter for a creamy lather or opting for hemp oil's moisturizing benefits enable you to design soaps that are not only kind to the environment but also luxurious in feel and function. Let's celebrate the journey of creating conscientious, cruelty-free soaps that stand as a testament to your commitment to a more sustainable lifestyle.

Plant-Based Soap Recipes

These are a fantastic way to create luxurious, eco-friendly soaps that align with vegan and palm-free principles. These recipes focus on using ingredients derived exclusively from plants, ensuring that your soap creations are both kind to the environment and gentle on the skin. By emphasizing the use of oils, butters, and botanicals, you'll craft soaps that are not only nourishing but also sustainable.

One of the most exciting aspects of plant-based soapmaking is the exploration of different oils and butters. Oils such as olive, coconut, and sunflower offer various benefits, from moisturizing properties to rich lather. Butters like shea, cocoa, and mango bring their own unique textures and nourishing qualities. When combined, these ingredients can create soaps that cater to a diverse range of skin types and preferences.

Let's dive into an example of a simple yet nourishing plant-based soap recipe: the classic olive and coconut oil soap. Start by measuring out your ingredients: 16 ounces of olive oil, 16 ounces of coconut oil, 6.3 ounces of sodium hydroxide (lye), and 15.2 ounces of distilled water. Following proper safety measures, carefully mix the lye into the water and allow it to cool. Once both the lye solution and oils are at a similar temperature, slowly mix them together. You'll know it's time to pour into molds when the mixture reaches 'trace,' the stage where it thickens to a pudding-like consistency.

A unique twist on the basic recipe is to replace some of the olive oil with avocado oil. Avocado oil, rich in vitamins A, D, and E, brings an extra nourishing factor to the soap. For this modified version, use 12 ounces of olive oil and add 4 ounces of avocado oil, keeping the rest of the ingredients the same. The emerald hue of avocado oil also imparts a subtle, natural color to your finished product.

For those who love experimenting with scents, essential oils are a game changer in plant-based soap recipes. Lavender and peppermint essential oils make a refreshing combination. Add 2 ounces of lavender and 1 ounce of peppermint essential oil to your soap mixture at trace. This blend not only smells delightful but also offers soothing and invigorating properties to the skin.

Essential Soaps

Incorporating herbs and botanicals elevates both the aesthetic and therapeutic qualities of your soaps. Consider a rosemary and mint soap infused with dried rosemary and peppermint leaves. Begin by mixing 16 ounces of coconut oil with 16 ounces of avocado oil, and add 15.2 ounces of distilled water and 6.3 ounces of lye. Once the mixture reaches trace, stir in 2 tablespoons of finely chopped dried rosemary and 1 tablespoon of dried peppermint leaves. Complement these botanicals by adding 1 ounce of rosemary essential oil and 1 ounce of peppermint essential oil.

Clays and other natural additives can also be used to enhance the texture and appearance of your plant-based soaps. French green clay, for instance, is known for its oil-absorbing properties and can give your soap a lovely green color. Try a green tea and French green clay soap by blending together 12 ounces of olive oil, 12 ounces of coconut oil, and 8 ounces of sweet almond oil. During the trace stage, add 2 tablespoons of French green clay and 2 ounces of green tea extract.

Plant-Based Soap Recipes also feature unique liquid alternatives that add another layer of nourishment. Aloe vera juice, for instance, can replace water in your recipe to provide extra soothing benefits. A simple recipe using aloe vera includes 14 ounces of coconut oil, 14 ounces of olive oil, 7 ounces of shea butter, and instead of 15.2 ounces of water, use 15.2 ounces of aloe vera juice. The result is a soap that's not only moisturizing but also calming for sensitive skin.

Texture variations can make your soaps even more interesting. Oatmeal is a fantastic natural exfoliant suitable for all skin types. To create an oatmeal and lavender soap, use 12 ounces of olive oil, 12 ounces of coconut oil, and 12 ounces of shea butter. At trace, add 2 ounces of ground oatmeal and 2 ounces of lavender essential oil. The oatmeal provides gentle exfoliation, while the lavender essential oil adds a calming scent.

For those seeking a luxurious lather, castor oil is a valuable addition to your plant-based recipes. A recipe for a luscious lathering soap could include 10 ounces of olive oil, 10 ounces of coconut oil, 5 ounces of palm-free shortening, and 3 ounces of castor oil. Add 2 ounces of cedarwood essential oil and 2 ounces of tea tree essential oil at trace for an earthy, refreshing aroma.

Every plant-based soap recipe can be tailored to your personal preferences. Experiment by mixing and matching different oils, butters, essential oils, and botanicals. Not only will this create a unique and personalized product, but it will also keep the soapmaking process exciting and fulfilling. Creating plant-based soaps ensures that your craft is aligned with sustainable and ethical practices, making it better for the planet and your skin. Happy soapmaking!

Remember, these recipes are just starting points. Feel free to get creative with additional additives such as activated charcoal, turmeric, or even finely ground coffee for exfoliation. Observation and experimentation are key to finding your perfect blend. Through practice, you'll discover the joys and benefits of creating plant-based soap that's as beautiful as it is beneficial.

Sustainable Alternatives to Palm Oil

These have become a significant focus for modern soapmakers, driven by the desire to create eco-friendly products. Palm oil, while popular for its excellent properties in soapmaking, is associated with severe environmental issues such as deforestation and habitat destruction. It's crucial to explore other options that not only maintain the quality of your soaps but also contribute positively to the environment.

One prominent alternative to palm oil is *olive oil*. Known for its moisturizing and gentle properties, olive oil produces a soap with a creamy lather that's perfect for sensitive skin. It's widely available and, if sourced thoughtfully, it can be a very sustainable option. Olive oil is hydrating and nourishing, rich in vitamins and antioxidants which are beneficial for all skin types. Additionally, it supports a slow-trace time during soapmaking, giving you ample time to work on intricate designs and patterns if you're contemplating a more artistic approach.

Another great substitute is *shea butter*. This luxurious fat, derived from the nuts of the African shea tree, is packed with vitamins A and E and offers unparalleled moisturizing benefits. Shea butter produces a hard, long-lasting bar of soap that's wonderfully conditioning. Sustainable shea butter is often harvested by women's cooperatives, supporting both the environment and the community.

Similarly, *cocoa butter* is an excellent choice for palm oil replacement. Known for its firm consistency and subtle chocolate aroma, cocoa butter imparts a rich emollient quality to soaps. It's ideal for creating luxurious bars that nurture dry skin. Sourcing fair-trade or organic cocoa butter can further ensure that your soapmaking is not only palm-free but also ethically conscious.

Coconut oil is another viable palm oil alternative that's beloved in the soapmaking community. It contributes to a bar's hardness and produces a fluffy, bubbly lather. Coconut oil is excellent for cleansing, though it can be drying if used in high quantities. A balanced recipe will counteract this, perhaps with the inclusion of other moisturizing fats like olive oil or shea butter. To ensure sustainability, look for coconut oil that's ethically sourced and certified organic.

Babassu oil provides a standout replacement for palm oil due to its similar fatty acid profile. Harvested from the fruit of the Babassu palm in Brazil, it's excellent for creating a hard bar with a creamy lather. It has a lightweight and non-greasy feel which makes it a favorite for those seeking an alternative to coconut oil. Importantly, the harvest process for babassu oil often supports local communities, making it a more sustainable and ethical choice.

For soapmakers looking to venture into unique oils, *rice bran oil* presents an intriguing option. Abundant in antioxidants, rice bran oil extends the shelf life of the soap, which is a valuable trait for any small business owner. It produces a rich, creamy lather and is highly moisturizing. Sourced from the hard outer layer of rice, it also supports agricultural sustainability.

Sunflower oil adds another versatile alternative to the mix. High in linoleic acid, this oil helps maintain the skin's barrier and reduces water loss, making for an incredibly hydrating soap. Sunflower oil also supports local agriculture in many regions, making it a sustainable choice when sourced from organic or small-scale farms.

Another fascinating option is *hemp seed oil*. Renowned for its unique fatty acid profile and impressive conditioning properties, hemp seed oil is both soothing and moisturizing. It's a more expensive option but well worth it for the quality it imparts to the soap. Sustainable hemp farming practices also contribute to soil health, making it a holistic alternative.

Additionally, it's worth considering *jojoba oil*, which technically is a liquid wax. This oil closely mimics the skin's natural sebum, providing deep moisture without feeling overly greasy. Jojoba oil is sustainable and usually grown with fewer pesticides, making it an excellent eco-friendly alternative. It adds luxurious conditioning properties to soap, yielding a bar that's both gentle and nurturing.

While experimenting with these alternatives, remember that creating a balanced soap recipe involves understanding the characteristics of each oil. A mix of hard and soft oils, for example, often provides the ideal balance of hardness, lather, and skin conditioning. Begin with small batches to refine your formulations, and use online calculators to perfect the ratios for optimum saponification and superfatting.

It's also important to support sustainable agriculture and ethical sourcing practices. When shopping for soapmaking supplies, seek out suppliers who are transparent about their sourcing and committed to environmental stewardship. Look for certifications like Fair Trade, USDA Organic, or RSPO (Roundtable on Sustainable Palm Oil) for palm replacements and other oils and butters.

Your choice to switch from palm oil to sustainable alternatives underlines a commitment that goes beyond crafting beautiful soaps. It embodies a growing movement toward environmental responsibility and ethical living. With every soap bar created from these sustainable alternatives, you contribute to a healthier planet, promoting biodiversity and supporting fair practices within the agricultural community.

As you continue your soapmaking journey, let your creativity and conscience guide you. Embrace the rich variety of nature's bounty in your formulations. Your artisanal soaps will not only stand out for their quality and distinctiveness but also tell a story of sustainability and mindful living. This is the kind of legacy that resonates with customers and inspires fellow crafters alike.

Chapter 15: Speciality Soaps and Techniques

Welcome to the delightful world of specialty soaps, where creativity and functionality go hand in hand. This chapter dives into advanced soapmaking techniques that elevate your soap game, introducing you to shampoo bars and conditioner soaps that cleanse and nourish your hair without the environmental footprint of plastic bottles. You'll also learn to craft luxurious shaving soaps that provide a smooth glide and superior lather, essential for a close, comfortable shave. Want to add an exfoliating kick to your routine? Scrub bars combine the benefits of soap with natural exfoliants, leaving your skin polished and refreshed. Each of these specialty soaps requires its own set of techniques and formulations, but the effort is well worth it. By mastering these, you're not just making soap; you're creating targeted, high-quality products that cater to specific needs and preferences. So, roll up your sleeves and let your soapmaking skills shine in this exciting foray into specialty soaps!

Shampoo Bars and Conditioner Soaps

Shampoo and conditioner soaps are an exciting frontier in the quest for natural, sustainable hair care. Whether you're a seasoned soapmaker or just getting started, these specialized bars can revolutionize your shower routine while reducing plastic waste. The beauty of creating your own shampoo bars and conditioner soaps lies in the customization options they offer. You can tailor each batch to suit specific hair types and needs, making these products not only eco-friendly but also highly effective.

First, let's talk about *why* you might want to make shampoo bars instead of sticking with conventional liquid shampoos. For one, shampoo bars are incredibly travel-friendly. No more worrying about TSA liquid limits or messy spills in your suitcase. Plus, they're more concentrated than their liquid counterparts. A single bar can last much longer than a bottle of shampoo, providing better value for money. Given their solid form, these bars also eliminate the need for plastic bottles, making them a more sustainable option for eco-conscious consumers.

Creating shampoo bars starts with choosing the right ingredients. You'll need oils and butters that nourish the scalp and hair without making it greasy. Popular choices include coconut oil for its lathering properties, olive oil for moisture, and castor oil to boost hair growth. For additional conditioning benefits, you can add shea butter or cocoa butter. Be mindful of the oil-to-lye ratio; you want to ensure the final product is neither too harsh nor too soft on the scalp.

Once you've selected your base oils, it's time to consider other beneficial additives. Essential oils play a significant role in providing both therapeutic and aromatic benefits. Lavender and rosemary essential oils, for instance, are excellent for scalp health and can help in reducing dandruff. Peppermint oil can invigorate the scalp and promote hair growth, while chamomile is soothing and ideal for sensitive skin.

Adding herbal infusions to your shampoo bars further heightens their appeal. Infused water or oil derived from herbs like nettle, horsetail, and calendula can provide additional scalp-nourishing benefits. These herbs can be steeped in the water phase of your soapmaking process or infused in your oils. You can also incorporate dried herb powders directly into the soap mixture for a more textured final product.

Conditioner soaps often get overlooked but can be just as transformative. While shampoo bars focus on cleansing and scalp health, conditioner soaps aim to replenish moisture and detangle hair. Typically, they have a higher concentration of conditioning butters and oils. For instance, avocado oil is perfect for deep conditioning, while jojoba oil closely mimics the scalp's natural sebum, making it highly effective at balancing oil production. Incorporating ingredients like aloe vera can provide additional hydration and soothe any scalp irritation.

To enhance the conditioning effect, you might also consider adding specific proteins like silk or oat protein. These proteins can strengthen hair shafts and provide a smoother, shinier appearance. Meanwhile, honey and glycerin can serve as humectants, drawing moisture into the hair and keeping it hydrated for longer periods.

The process of making shampoo bars and conditioner soaps is similar to traditional cold process soap but with a few key differences. For one, you may want to use a higher superfat percentage. Superfatting means you leave more unsaponified oils in your soap, which can add additional moisturizing properties. Typically, shampoo bars benefit from a superfat percentage of around 5-7%, while conditioner bars might go a bit higher, up to 10%.

One crucial consideration when formulating these products is pH level. Hair and scalp have a natural pH of around 4.5 to 5.5, which is slightly acidic. Traditional soap is alkaline, with a pH around 9-10. To balance this, you might consider adding citric acid to your formulation. A small amount can help lower the pH, making the final product more compatible with your scalp's natural environment.

Proper curing is vital for both shampoo and conditioner bars. Allow the bars to cure for at least 4-6 weeks to ensure they are firm and long-lasting. This curing time also helps to neutralize the pH further, making the bars gentler on your scalp. Store them in a dry, ventilated area and turn them occasionally to promote even curing.

Finally, let's not forget the aesthetic and sensory experience of using these hair care bars. Adding natural colorants like spirulina, turmeric, or indigo powder can make each bar visually inviting. Embedding dried flowers or herbs on the surface can add a touch of elegance. For fragrance, blend essential oils to create a signature scent that makes your daily shower feel luxurious and spa-like.

In summary, **shampoo bars and conditioner soaps** combine the joys of soapmaking with the practical benefits of hair care. They offer a customizable, eco-friendly alternative to commercial products, reducing your plastic footprint while catering to your unique hair needs. Whether you're looking to create these bars for personal use or to expand your small business offerings, the potential for creativity and effectiveness is immense.

With every batch you make, you contribute to a more sustainable future while indulging in the artistry of crafting nourishing, beneficial products for everyday use. Dive into your soapmaking with confidence, knowing that each bar you forge will bring you one step closer to not just cleaner hair, but a cleaner planet too.

Shaving Soaps and Scrub Bars

These often get overlooked in the vast world of soapmaking, but they're an essential niche worth mastering. Crafting these unique soaps not only broadens your skill set but also introduces you to a different kind of luxurious, functional product that your skin will love. Whether you're interested in making a rich, creamy lather for an ultrasmooth shave or a scrub bar that gently exfoliates the skin, there's a wealth of knowledge to dive into.

Let's start with shaving soaps. When creating a shaving soap, the goal is to produce a stable, creamy lather that provides plenty of slip for a razor to glide effortlessly over the skin. This means focusing on ingredients that contribute to both lather and conditioning. A good shaving soap typically includes a higher percentage of stearic acid, which helps to create a thick, rich foam. Beef tallow, palm oil, and mango butter are excellent sources of stearic acid and will lend that desired creaminess. Additionally, castor oil can enhance the lather while coconut oil provides cleansing and bubbly characteristics.

The process for making shaving soap involves much of what you're already familiar with if you've done cold process soapmaking. However, tweaking the ratios and ingredients is crucial. For instance, you might consider including bentonite clay for its slip properties, which allows the razor to glide smoothly without nicks or irritation. Furthermore, adding glycerin can boost the soap's moisturizing qualities, ensuring that skin feels hydrated and nourished post-shave.

To create the perfect shaving soap, it's essential to have a stable formula. Start with a base recipe and adjust according to your needs. Here's a simple starter recipe:

- Olive Oil - 25%
- Coconut Oil - 30%
- Castor Oil - 10%
- Palm Oil - 20%
- Beef Tallow - 15%
- Bentonite Clay - 2 tablespoons per pound of oils
- Glycerin - 5% of the total oils

This recipe should give you a rich, luxurious shaving soap that holds up well under use. Feel free to experiment with different additives and essential oil blends. A popular scent combination for shaving soaps includes peppermint and tea tree oil, which offers a refreshing and invigorating experience.

Scrub Bars, on the other hand, are about achieving the perfect balance between exfoliation and moisturizing. The aim here is to remove dead skin cells while providing nourishment to keep skin smooth and soft. When it comes to scrub bars, the choice of exfoliant is key. Some popular exfoliants include ground coffee, oats, sugar, and poppy seeds. Each has its unique texture and benefits.

Scrub bars can be crafted using either cold or hot process methods. Regardless of the method, you'll start with a base soap recipe. A good starting point is a recipe rich in moisturizing oils like olive, shea butter, and sweet almond oil. Here's a basic scrub bar recipe to get you going:

- Olive Oil - 40%
- Coconut Oil - 30%
- Shea Butter - 10%
- Sweet Almond Oil - 10%
- Castor Oil - 10%
- Oatmeal - 2 tablespoons per pound of oils

Incorporate your chosen exfoliant during trace, which helps the particles remain well-distributed throughout the soap. If you're using delicate exfoliants like oats or coffee grounds, it's best to minimize their concentration to avoid being too abrasive on the skin. For more robust exfoliants, like seeds or pumice, you can afford to use a heavier hand, but always test a small batch first.

Beyond the ingredients, it's important to consider the intended ambience and experience of the scrub bar. Essential oils can transform a simple scrub into an aromatherapeutic experience. For instance, a blend of lavender and eucalyptus can be both soothing and invigorating, perfect for an energizing morning scrub.

Once you have your formula locked down, the challenge will be presentation. Shaving soaps can be poured into molds that create a puck shape, which fits nicely into shaving bowls. For scrub bars, consider molds that emphasize the exfoliating feature, like textured bars or loaves that you can cut into chunky, hand-friendly pieces.

Another aspect to consider is color. Natural colorants, such as clays or activated charcoal, can add hues that align with the soap's purpose. For example, a charcoal scrub bar not only looks appealing but also utilizes charcoal's purifying properties. Similarly, rose clay can lend a pink tint and add to the soap's skin-smoothing benefits.

Advanced techniques can also be applied to both shaving soaps and scrub bars. Layering, swirling, or embedding exfoliating ingredients can add visual appeal and differentiate your products. Imagine a scrub bar with delicate flower petals or a shaving soap with a two-tone swirl that catches the eye.

Finally, product longevity is key. For shaving soaps, encourage users to let the soap dry between uses to extend its lifespan. As for scrub bars, ensuring even distribution of scrub materials will help maintain efficacy down to the last sliver.

Incorporating these advanced details will set your shaving soaps and scrub bars apart from commercially available products. Remember, you have the unique advantage of customizing every element, from ingredients to design, making each creation a true embodiment of artisan craftsmanship.

Now, with your shaving and scrub bars perfected, you're well on your way to mastering the nuanced world of specialty soaps. Keep experimenting and refining your recipes. Your creativity is the only limit, and the delight of creating something both beautiful and functional will undoubtedly pay off, enhancing not just the product but the entire experience for the user.

The satisfaction of crafting these niche products is unparalleled. As you delve deeper into shaving soaps and scrub bars, you'll discover that each batch, each experiment, brings you closer to mastering the fine art of soapmaking. So, get your tools ready and embrace the challenge – your next best soap awaits.

Chapter 16:
Soap for Babies and Sensitive Skin

Crafting soap for babies and sensitive skin is a joyful and deeply gratifying endeavor that calls for simplicity and purity. When formulating these gentle soaps, opt for ingredients that are known for their soothing and hypoallergenic properties, such as olive oil, coconut oil, and shea butter. Avoid harsh fragrances and colorants, favoring instead the natural hues and subtle, calming scents provided by chamomile and calendula. These ingredients not only cleanse but also nourish delicate skin, providing essential moisture and protection. Unscented options are highly recommended to minimize the risk of irritation. By focusing on creating mild, nurturing soaps, you're ensuring a tender touch for the most sensitive skin types and offering peace of mind for parents. Embrace this opportunity to blend simplicity with effectiveness, resulting in creations that are as kind to the Earth as they are to the skin.

Gentle Formulas and Hypoallergenic Ingredients

Gentle and hypoallergenic ingredients are like a soothing lullaby for your skin, especially for those with delicate or sensitive skin types. Creating soap that is not only effective but also gentle requires careful selection and preparation of ingredients. By focusing on hypoallergenic ingredients, we can craft products that minimize irritation and provide soothing relief to sensitive areas.

Essential Soaps

To start, understanding what makes a soap "gentle" is crucial. Generally, it's about the balance between cleansing and moisturizing properties, followed by the incorporation of ingredients known for their soothing capabilities. Traditional soap formulations often contain synthetic fragrances and detergents that can be harsh. In contrast, natural soapmaking emphasizes botanical ingredients and natural emollients that promote skin health without irritation.

An important factor in formulating gentle soaps is choosing the right base oils. Oils like olive oil, avocado oil, and sweet almond oil are renowned for their moisturizing and nourishing qualities. These oils provide essential fatty acids and vitamins that support skin barrier function. Olive oil, in particular, has been used for centuries and is famed for its gentle, conditioning properties. Combining these oils can create a rich, creamy lather that's kind to sensitive skin.

Beyond oils, the inclusion of butters such as shea and cocoa butter can significantly enhance the soap's gentleness. Shea butter, for example, is packed with vitamins A and E, and provides deep hydration. It's also anti-inflammatory, making it an excellent choice for reducing redness and irritation. When these butters are incorporated into soap recipes, they contribute to a luxurious feel and long-lasting moisture.

Another key consideration is the use of hypoallergenic ingredients, which are less likely to cause allergic reactions. Goat milk is a fantastic option here. Rich in fatty acids and vitamins, goat milk offers gentle exfoliation and deep moisturization, making it ideal for sensitive skin formulations. It's also known for its mild pH, which aligns closely with that of human skin, reducing the risk of irritation.

Oatmeal is an ingredient that deserves special mention. It's often hailed for its soothing, anti-inflammatory properties. Finely ground oatmeal can be added to soap recipes to create a mild exfoliant that gently removes dead skin cells while calming irritated skin. Oatmeal has been used for ages in treatments for various skin conditions like eczema and psoriasis, highlighting its effectiveness.

While formulating gentle soaps, it's also vital to consider the potential allergens. Common allergens in soapmaking can include nut oils, gluten-containing grains, and certain botanical extracts. Being mindful of these ingredients and opting for hypoallergenic alternatives ensures that your soaps cater to a broader audience, including those with allergies.

Essential oils can also play a role in gentle soap formulations, but with caution. Though they are natural, some essential oils can be potent and irritating to sensitive skin. Lavender and chamomile essential oils are excellent choices for their calming and anti-inflammatory properties. Lavender, for instance, not only adds a soothing fragrance but also promotes skin healing. Chamomile is another wonderfully gentle oil that helps calm skin irritation and redness.

Hydrosols or floral waters are a less concentrated alternative to essential oils and can be used to impart a mild, soothing fragrance to soaps. Rose water and cucumber water are both gentle and beneficial for the skin, offering hydration and a subtle scent without the intensity of essential oils.

In the realm of hypoallergenic soapmaking, less is often more. Limiting the number of ingredients can reduce the risk of skin reactions. Simple soaps with just a few, well-chosen ingredients can be profoundly effective and gentle. A basic recipe might include just olive oil, goat milk, and a touch of oatmeal. This minimalist approach ensures that each ingredient serves a purpose and contributes to the overall gentleness of the soap.

It's also essential to consider the role of water in soap formulations. Distilled water is typically used to avoid the impurities found in tap water that could cause skin irritation. This extra step is particularly important when crafting soaps for sensitive skin, ensuring the soap is as pure and gentle as possible.

Understanding the saponification process is also crucial. Fully saponified soap should ideally have no residual lye, which can be harsh and irritating. Proper curing times allow for any excess lye to neutralize, resulting in a mild and safe end product. Ensuring a thorough saponification process, coupled with a robust curing period, contributes significantly to the gentleness of the soap.

Superfatting is another technique worth mentioning. By leaving a portion of the oils unsaponified, the final soap retains more of the oils' moisturizing properties. This is pivotal in formulations for sensitive skin, where the extra conditioning can make a substantial difference. Superfatting at around 5-8% is typically effective in creating a moisturizing, gentle soap.

Cold process soapmaking is often preferred for creating gentle and hypoallergenic soaps since it allows for greater control over the ingredients and their properties. The lower temperatures preserve the integrity of the oils and butters, ensuring they retain their beneficial properties. Hot process soapmaking can also be gentle, but it requires careful temperature control and timing to avoid overcooking the ingredients.

Whether you're crafting for infants or adults with sensitive skin, testing your soap is a crucial step. Patch testing on a small area of skin can help identify any potential irritants. Encouraging your audience to use this method will provide peace of mind and ensure the soap's gentleness before full use.

Formulating gentle and hypoallergenic soaps doesn't just benefit those with sensitive skin; it's a testament to the care and thought put into your soapmaking practice. By selecting gentle base ingredients, mindful of potential allergens, and understanding the intricacies of saponification and superfatting, you're well on your way to creating soothing, skin-loving products. Embrace the simplicity and purity of these formulations. Your customers, whether it's family, friends, or loyal clientele, will thank you for the kindness and thoughtfulness poured into each bar.

Now that you've grasped the essentials of gentle formulas and hypoallergenic ingredients, let's explore how to craft unscented and soothing soaps in the next subsection. These recipes will build on what you've learned here, offering even more options for creating the gentlest soap possible.

Unscented and Soothing Soaps

These offer a gentle haven for those with sensitive skin or fragrance sensitivities. By removing essential oils and fragrances, you focus on the core aspects of soapmaking—nourishing ingredients, gentle cleansers, and soothing additives that harmonize with the skin. This sub-section will guide you through the essentials of crafting unscented soaps that soothe and nourish, turning each bar into a miniature spa experience.

Creating unscented soap doesn't mean sacrificing the benefits and luxurious feel of natural bars. On the contrary, unscented soaps can be exceptionally enriching when formulated with the right mix of oils, butters, and botanicals. Think of ingredients like oat milk, chamomile, and calendula which offer a calming touch to the soap, perfect for anyone looking to avoid potential irritants commonly found in synthetic fragrances.

Start by selecting base oils that are known for their moisturizing properties. Oils such as olive, coconut, and avocado offer a rich, creamy lather while providing essential nutrients and vitamins. Combine them with butters like shea and cocoa, which add an extra layer of hydration and luxury to the final product. Balancing your oil and butter ratios ensures a soap that is not only soothing but also effective in cleansing the skin without stripping its natural oils.

Remember, even without aromatic essential oils, botanicals play an instrumental role in adding subtle characteristics to your soap. Chamomile and calendula petals, when infused in oils, can lend their anti-inflammatory and skin-soothing properties. These herbs are well-known for their gentle action, making them ideal for a calming bath experience. Simply infuse your chosen herbs in your base oil before adding it to your soap mixture to capture their beneficial properties.

A key aspect of unscented soapmaking is ensuring that the pH level is carefully maintained. This helps in producing a bar that is kind to even the most delicate skin types. While the natural process of saponification generally results in a balanced pH, it's good practice to test your soap to make sure it falls within a skin-friendly range, typically between 7 and 10 on the pH scale. Overly alkaline soaps can be harsh, while those too acidic may not cleanse effectively.

- Olive Oil: Moisturizing and gentle, rich in antioxidants.
- Coconut Oil: Adds lather, has antimicrobial properties.
- Avocado Oil: Packed with vitamins A, D, and E.
- Shea Butter: Deeply nourishing and moisturizing.
- Cocoa Butter: Adds firmness and hydration.

When working with sensitive skin, it's important to consider the curing time of your soap. Allowing your soap to cure for at least four to six weeks will ensure all lye has been converted, resulting in a mild bar. During this time, water evaporates from the soap, making it harder and longer-lasting. Patience is key here; a fully cured bar of soap is less likely to cause irritation and lasts significantly longer in the shower.

Texture and appearance are other aspects you can play with to make your unscented soap more attractive. Natural additives like oatmeal, which gently exfoliates, can also enhance the soothing qualities of your soap. Goat milk adds a creamy texture that's luxuriously moisturizing, making your soap a pampering treat. The unscented approach allows these natural ingredients to shine, both in their benefits and their pure, unadulterated beauty.

Oatmeal, as an additive, deserves a special mention. Known for its anti-inflammatory properties, it's perfect for soothing conditions like eczema and psoriasis. Oatmeal not only adds a gentle exfoliating quality to the soap but also imparts a creamy feel that enhances the moisturizing experience. Use finely ground oatmeal for a smooth finish or rolled oats for a textural contrast. Either way, incorporating oatmeal transforms a simple soap bar into a soothing, healing experience.

For those who would like to add a touch of color without introducing potential irritants, natural clays are an excellent option. Clays like kaolin or rose clay offer subtle hues while adding detoxifying properties to the soap. They gently draw out impurities from the skin, making them a fantastic addition without compromising the gentle nature of your soap. Just remember to add the clays sparingly, as too much can alter the soap's consistency.

1. Finely Ground Oatmeal: Soothes and gently exfoliates.
2. Goat Milk: Adds creaminess and extra hydration.
3. Kaolin Clay: Detoxifies and gives a soft texture.
4. Calendula: Offers calming and healing properties.
5. Chamomile: Provides anti-inflammatory benefits.

When crafting unscented soaps, the process may seem simple at first glance, but it's an art to balance the ingredients perfectly to deliver a wholesome experience. Leveraging the natural properties of oils and butters, coupled with soothing botanical infusions, each bar of soap can be a luxurious, skin-nourishing gift to yourself or others. For those who suffer from sensitive skin or prefer to avoid any fragrances, these unscented soaps become a sanctuary for the senses.

Embrace the creativity that comes with formulating unscented and soothing soaps. The absence of strong scents allows the inherent qualities of your chosen ingredients to take center stage. Whether you're indulging in the creamy lather of a shea butter base or the gentle exfoliation from oatmeal, each ingredient has a purpose and offers a unique benefit. The key lies in understanding the properties of what you put into your soap and how they interact to create a balanced and effective product.

Imagine the satisfaction of gifting loved ones a bar of unscented soap that you've crafted specifically for their skincare needs. The thought and care behind the selection of ingredients will not go unnoticed. These soaps are often more than just a cleansing tool; they become a symbol of care and mindfulness. And for those looking to turn this hobby into a small business, unscented soaps cater to a niche market, appealing especially to customers with allergies or sensitive skin.

Consider adding a luxurious touch by finely milling your soap batter, ensuring a smooth and consistent texture in each bar. This technique can elevate the user experience, making every wash feel indulgent. Pair this with a beautiful, simple packaging, focusing on the purity and quality of your soap, and you've got a product that stands out in a crowded market.

In summary, crafting **Unscented and Soothing Soaps** requires thoughtfulness and a deep understanding of the ingredients involved. By focusing on skin-nourishing oils, soothing botanicals, and gentle additives, you can create soaps that are perfect for those with sensitive skin or allergies. The beauty of unscented soaps lies in their simplicity, highlighting the essence of natural soapmaking and offering a pure, holistic approach to skincare. Enjoy the journey of soapmaking, combining creativity and care to produce what could very well become a staple in the world of

Chapter 17: Themed and Seasonal Soapmaking

Dive into the world of themed and seasonal soapmaking, where creativity takes center stage, allowing you to tailor your soap creations to match any occasion or time of year. Whether whipping up festive holiday bars adorned with glittery swirls and warm spiced scents or crafting refreshing summer soaps imbued with citrus and floral notes, the possibilities are endless. Seasonal soapmaking not only keeps your crafting experience fresh and exciting but also provides an excellent opportunity for those looking to market their soaps. Customers are often drawn to unique, limited-edition products that capture the essence of a particular season or celebration. By aligning your soap designs, colors, and fragrances with various holidays and seasonal moods, you can create an irresistible lineup that resonates with every soap aficionado's desire for variety and novelty while also celebrating the natural cycles of the year.

Holiday and Celebration Soaps

This category of soaps holds a magical place in the world of soapmaking, giving you endless possibilities to create themed soaps that bring joy and evoke memories. Special occasions are the perfect excuse to experiment with colors, fragrances, and decorative elements that highlight the spirit of the season. From Christmas to Halloween, each holiday provides opportunities to infuse your soaps with unique characteristics that encapsulate the essence of celebration.

The first step in crafting Holiday and Celebration Soaps is to decide which holiday or event you're targeting. Once you've pinpointed your focus, the process becomes much simpler and truly enjoyable. For instance, Christmas soaps can feature classic red and green colors, or incorporate festive fragrances like peppermint and pine. On the other hand, Halloween soaps might take on the eerie glow of purples and black, scented with rich spices that hint at autumn's arrival. The sky is the limit when you're allowing your soaps to tell a story of celebration.

Choosing the right colors for your holiday soaps is crucial because colors are intrinsically linked with festive feelings. For Christmas, think green for Christmas trees or red and white for candy canes. Valentine's Day practically begs for shades of red and pink, often swirled together in heart-shaped molds. Easter brings pastels to mind, while patriotic holidays call for red, white, and blue. For all occasions, natural colorants like mica powders or clays can provide vivid, safe hues that enhance the visual appeal of your creations.

One of the most distinguishing features of holiday soaps is their scent. Essential oils play a significant role in bringing the aroma of the season into your soap bars. Cinnamon, nutmeg, and clove essential oils can give a warm, inviting fragrance to Thanksgiving-themed soaps. Meanwhile, lavender can evoke a sense of peace and renewal that's perfect for New Year's. Experiment with blending different essential oils to create a unique scent profile that captures the spirit of each holiday.

Beyond color and scent, adding textures and decorations can further elevate your holiday soaps. Soap embeds, created using melt and pour soap base, can range from small stars and snowflakes to pumpkins and hearts, depending on the occasion. These small touches, when integrated into larger bars, can create a layered experience that makes soap almost too pretty to use. Glitter, botanicals, and even small ornaments can be safely embedded in the soap to add a touch of whimsy and delight.

Let's not forget about the molds! Specific molds can help create instantly recognizable shapes that enhance the festive theme of your soaps. Silicone molds in the shapes of Christmas trees, Easter eggs, or autumn leaves make for an excellent presentation. These molds can handle the cold process and melt and pour methods alike, allowing you the flexibility to experiment with different techniques while maintaining the holiday theme.

Packaging is another essential aspect of Holiday and Celebration Soaps. The presentation makes a significant impact, especially if you're planning to give these soaps as gifts or sell them in a market setting. Eco-friendly kraft paper with festive ribbons, reusable tins, or even biodegradable shrink wrap can elevate the appearance of your holiday soaps. Labels can convey the story behind each soap, listing ingredients and sharing a heartfelt message, adding a personal touch that resonates with the recipient.

The importance of sustainability and eco-friendliness in your soapmaking practices cannot be overstated, particularly during the holidays when consumerism is at its peak. Opt for sustainably sourced ingredients, avoid synthetic fragrances, and use recyclable or compostable packaging materials. This not only contributes positively to the environment but also differentiates your soaps as mindful, responsible, and high-quality products that stand above mass-produced options.

Creating themed sets of soaps for holidays and celebrations can also be an exciting way to showcase a variety of designs and scents. A gift set for Christmas might include a peppermint-scented soap shaped like a candy cane, a tree-shaped bar with pine fragrance, and a star-shaped soap with a cinnamon and clove blend. Sets can be a fantastic approach to offer a full sensory experience and make an excellent gift choice for friends and family or an impressive collection for market sales.

Incorporating personalized elements into your holiday soaps can make these creations even more special. Initials, custom messages, and bespoke fragrances can transform a simple bar of soap into a cherished keepsake. This can be particularly impactful for weddings, baby showers, or milestone birthdays where guests expect a memorable souvenir.

Holiday and Celebration Soaps are not just confined to traditional celebrations; they can also commemorate personal milestones and achievements. Think of graduation soaps in school colors, anniversary soaps with scents that bring back wedding day memories, or new baby soaps in baby blues and pinks with calming chamomile and lavender scents. The emotional tie these soaps can create makes them meaningful gifts that go beyond their functional purpose.

For soapmaking enthusiasts who are looking to turn their hobby into a profitable venture, holiday soaps offer an exceptional opportunity. Themed soaps are highly marketable, particularly during peak holiday seasons when consumers are in search of unique, homemade gifts. Limited edition holiday collections can create a sense of urgency and exclusivity, encouraging customers to purchase before they miss out. Marketing seasons like "Christmas in July" can also help stretch these opportunities throughout the year.

In terms of marketing strategies, social media plays a vital role in showcasing your beautiful holiday soaps. Platforms like Instagram and Pinterest are excellent for sharing visually stunning photos of your creations, offering a glimpse into your creative process and allowing you to engage directly with your audience. Consider creating tutorial videos or behind-the-scene glimpses that show the making of your holiday soaps, further fostering a connection with your customers.

Overall, the adventure of making Holiday and Celebration Soaps is a wondrous exploration of creativity, emotion, and craftsmanship. Every season and every occasion bring new inspiration and new opportunities to craft something truly special. Whether you're making these soaps for personal enjoyment, as heartfelt gifts, or for sale, each bar becomes a storyteller, capturing the essence of the moment and spreading joy to all who receive it.

Creating a Seasonal Soap Line

This idea could be one of the most exciting and creatively fulfilling endeavors in your soapmaking journey. Seasonality not only allows you to tap into the bounty of nature's seasonal offerings, but it also gives your customers something new and fresh to look forward to throughout the year. In this section, we'll explore how to harness the essence of each season to craft soaps that are not only functional but infused with the spirit and fragrances of the time of year.

First off, think about what makes each season special. What colors, scents, and ingredients come to mind when you think of spring, summer, fall, and winter? For example, spring could bring to mind blooming flowers and greenery, while fall might remind you of cozy spices and pumpkins. Understanding these associations will help guide your ingredient choices, making your seasonal soaps more appealing and evocative.

Spring is a time of renewal and growth. For your spring soap line, consider using herbs and flowers like lavender, chamomile, and calendula. These ingredients not only add visual appeal but also contribute to the overall skin-loving properties of your soaps. Essential oils such as geranium, rosemary, and eucalyptus can bring a fresh, uplifting aroma that complements the vibrant, rejuvenating nature of spring. You might also want to experiment with pastel colorants derived from natural sources, such as spirulina for a soft green or purple Brazilian clay for a lavender hue.

As we transition to summer, the spotlight shifts to bright, vibrant, and often tropical influences. Ingredients like coconut oil, aloe vera, and citrus peels can provide a cooling and refreshing sensation, perfect for hot summer days. Essential oils such as lime, sweet orange, and ylang-ylang can evoke a sense of beachside relaxation and sunny days. Don't shy away from bright, vivid colors often associated with summer; think oranges, yellows, and even pops of hot pink, made possible using turmeric, carrot juice, or rose clay.

Fall is the season of warmth and coziness. It's time to bring out the rich, earthy fragrances and deeper hues. Pumpkin puree, cinnamon, clove, and nutmeg can add not only wonderful fall scents but also beneficial properties, like gentle exfoliation and antibacterial effects. Essential oils such as patchouli, sandalwood, and cedarwood can add complexity and warmth to your scents, making your soap feel like a comforting hug. Think about adding exfoliants like ground oats or coffee grounds for a bit of texture and an added sense of indulgence.

Winter is a time for luxury and indulgence, a season to pamper and protect the skin from harsh elements. Ingredients like shea butter, cocoa butter, and goat milk can provide deep nourishment and hydration. For scent, consider essential oils such as peppermint, pine, and frankincense to evoke the crispness and festivity of the winter season. Deep, rich colors like dark greens, blues, and whites, derived from indigo powder and activated charcoal, can make your winter soaps stand out as holiday gifts or personal indulgence items.

Now that we have an idea of the key ingredients and scents to use for each season, it's crucial to think about how you'll present your seasonal soap line. Packaging, naming, and marketing all play significant roles in the success of your seasonal products. Use packaging materials that align with the season; for example, lightweight

Essential Soaps

and airy packaging for spring and summer, and more robust, cozy packaging for fall and winter. Naming your soaps to reflect the season can also enhance their appeal, such as "Lavender Bloom" for spring or "Winter Wonderland" for winter.

Marketing your seasonal soap line can be a fun and creative process. Use social media platforms to share the story behind each season's line, showing behind-the-scenes creation processes or explaining the benefits of the seasonal ingredients. Create anticipation by teasing upcoming releases and offering limited-time seasonal bundles. Engaging your audience with seasonal themes can increase excitement and drive sales.

Let's take a moment to consider how you can keep your seasonal soap line sustainable and eco-friendly. As the backdrop to everything you create, sustainability should always be at the forefront of your planning. Sourcing local, organic ingredients not only supports community agriculture but also reduces your carbon footprint. Consider using biodegradable packaging options, like recycled paper or compostable bags, which resonate well with eco-conscious consumers.

Creating a seasonal soap line can be a deeply rewarding experience. It allows you to continually innovate and refresh your product offerings, keeping your hobby or business dynamic and engaging. By thoughtfully selecting ingredients and carefully considering the aesthetics and fragrances of each soap, you can craft products that not only meet the needs of your customers but also bring a piece of each season into their daily lives.

In summary, creating a seasonal soap line involves more than just changing a few ingredients; it requires a deep understanding of the essence of each season and how to capture that in a bar of soap. It's about blending creativity with craftsmanship, and nature with nurture, to create products that not only cleanse but also tell a story.

And isn't telling stories through our crafts one of the most beautiful things we can do?

Now, it's your turn. Start dreaming up your seasonal soap lines and put your creativity to work with the endless inspiration that nature offers. You'll find that each season brings with it a unique palette of colors, scents, and ingredients that will not only enrich your soapmaking but also delight your senses and those of your customers. Happy soapmaking!

Chapter 18:
Packaging and Presentation

So, you've crafted your batch of beautiful, natural soap, infused with aromatic essential oils and skin-loving herbs. Now comes the crucial step of packaging and presentation, which not only protects your soaps but also enhances their appeal. Eco-friendly packaging options abound, from recycled paper wraps and compostable boxes to reusable tins and cloth bags that echo the sustainable ethos of your handcrafted creations. It's essential to adhere to labeling regulations, clearly listing ingredients, weight, and any pertinent safety information, ensuring that your customers know exactly what they're getting. Remember, the presentation is an art in itself—let your creativity shine through in design while maintaining an authentic, transparent connection with your audience. Effective packaging can elevate your soap from a simple product to an irresistible gift, turning first-time buyers into loyal fans.

Eco-Friendly Packaging Options

Offering eco-friendly packaging is a crucial consideration for any soapmaker who wants to integrate sustainability into their craft. As we develop our beautiful, natural soaps, the packaging we choose should reflect our commitment to the environment. Let's dive into several eco-friendly options that not only protect our soaps but also minimize our environmental footprint.

When it comes to packaging, one of the most accessible and eco-conscious materials is paper. Paper and cardboard are biodegradable, recyclable, and readily available. You can explore options like kraft paper or recycled cardboard boxes to give your soaps a rustic, natural look. Not only do they complement the aesthetic of handmade, natural soaps, but they also decompose quickly, reducing waste. For those of you who fancy a bit more creativity, consider using seed paper. This type of paper can be planted after use, resulting in beautiful flowers or herbs.

Another excellent choice is fabric. Fabric wraps, like muslin or cotton, can be reused and are biodegradable. They offer a charming, old-world style to your packaging that evokes a sense of craftsmanship and care. Wrapping your soaps in fabric not only looks aesthetically pleasing but also provides an extra layer of protection. You could even consider using upcycled fabric from old clothing or linens, adding a unique touch to each package. This not only reduces waste but also tells a story with each piece of fabric reused.

Jute and burlap are also fantastic materials to consider. These natural fibers are incredibly durable, biodegradable, and lend an earthy, rustic feel to your soap packaging. Small jute bags or burlap wraps can be used to package individual bars of soap or sets of soaps. They're great for gift packaging due to their sturdy structure and unique texture, which stands out in a market full of plastics.

For soapmakers looking to push the envelope, consider experimenting with biodegradable plastic alternatives. Products like PLA (Polylactic Acid) plastics, made from fermented plant starch (usually corn), offer an eco-friendly alternative to conventional plastics. They biodegrade under specific conditions and can be an excellent choice for those needing a more protective, plastic-like material.

Glass containers, though less common, offer a sturdy, reusable option for soap packaging. While they aren't biodegradable, glass can be recycled endlessly without losing quality. Moreover, glass jars or bottles can be repurposed by your customers, giving them a second life beyond their initial use. This makes glass a sustainable option worth considering, especially for liquid soaps or soap scrubs.

Beyond the material itself, consider the overall design and assembly of your packaging. Aim to minimize the use of tape, glue, and other non-biodegradable sealing methods. Simple folding techniques for boxes and wraps can eliminate the need for these adhesives. For example, a beautifully folded paper wrap can secure a bar of soap without any additional fasteners. Additionally, opt for natural twines or ribbons made of hemp or cotton instead of synthetic options.

Stickers and labels are another important component of packaging. Traditional paper stickers might include adhesive backs that aren't always eco-friendly. Instead, look into biodegradable labels with plant-based adhesives or simply print directly onto your packaging materials when possible. Another option is to use a rubber stamp with eco-friendly ink on kraft paper tags or directly onto fabric wraps.

To further minimize waste, consider adopting a zero-waste mindset during your packaging process. By designing packaging that can be reused or composted, you reduce the need for single-use materials. Moreover, encourage your customers to join you in these efforts by providing information on how they can reuse or properly dispose of the packaging.

If you run a soapmaking business, eco-friendly packaging isn't just a responsible choice—it can also be a compelling selling point. Displaying your commitment to sustainability can attract customers who value and support eco-conscious brands. Clearly communicate your packaging choices on your website, social media, and product labels. Sharing the story behind your packaging can build a deeper connection with your audience and differentiate your products in a crowded market.

Consider collaborating with local artists or craftsmen to create unique, artisanal packaging solutions that reflect your brand's values. Handmade boxes, fabric wraps with custom designs, or stamped labels can add a touch of personalization that mass-produced packaging simply can't offer. This not only supports local businesses but also enhances the overall presentation of your soaps.

Sourcing materials locally is another way to reduce the carbon footprint of your packaging. By choosing local suppliers, you cut down on transportation emissions and support the local economy. Plus, local materials are often more sustainable, as they haven't traveled long distances to reach you.

Lastly, remember that the journey to completely eco-friendly packaging is a progressive one. Experiment with different materials and designs to find what works best for your products and your values. Innovate, iterate, and continually seek out new ways to make your packaging more sustainable. Every small change adds up and makes a significant difference in the long run.

In conclusion, **Eco-Friendly Packaging Options** are an integral part of sustainable soapmaking. Whether you choose paper, fabric, jute, biodegradable plastics, or glass, your packaging choices reflect your commitment to the environment. By incorporating these options, you not only reduce your environmental impact but also connect with customers who share your values. Let's continue to prioritize eco-friendly practices and inspire others to do the same in every aspect of our soapmaking journey.

Labeling Regulations and Best Practices

Labeling your product plays a crucial role in the presentation and success of your handcrafted soaps. Whether you're making soaps for personal use, gifts, or selling them at farmers' markets and online, adhering to labeling regulations is non-negotiable. It's not just about following the law; clear, accurate labels can build trust with your customers, highlighting the transparency, quality, and benefits of your products.

First and foremost, you need to understand the legal requirements for labeling handmade soap, especially if you plan on selling your creations. In the United States, the Food and Drug Administration (FDA) has specific guidelines that all soapmakers must follow. According to FDA guidelines, a true soap must be primarily composed of alkali salts of fatty acids and be labeled as soap. If your soap contains synthetic detergents or claims to do things beyond just cleaning — like moisturizing or exfoliating — it might be considered a cosmetic or even a drug, both of which have stringent labeling rules.

The FDA requires that labels must include the identity of the product, the net weight of the product, and the name and address of the manufacturer. The identity of the product must plainly state that it's soap. For instance, you can simply label it as "Handmade Soap" or "Natural Soap." The net weight should be listed in both ounces and grams, giving your customers a clear idea of the amount of product they are purchasing.

A critical aspect often overlooked is the ingredient list. Even though soaps are exempt from the full ingredient disclosure requirements applicable to cosmetics, listing your ingredients can foster consumer trust and transparency. It's best practice to list ingredients in descending order of predominance, using their common names. For example, you might list "Olive Oil, Coconut Oil, Lye, Lavender Essential Oil" instead of their chemical names. This makes it easier for customers to understand what's in the soap and helps those with allergies avoid potential irritants.

Moreover, if you're selling your soap as a cosmetic, the labeling needs to follow stricter guidelines. This includes a full disclosure of all ingredients, listed by their International Nomenclature of Cosmetic Ingredients (INCI) names. For example, instead of "Coconut Oil," you'd list "Cocos Nucifera Oil." Failure to adhere can result in penalties or your product being removed from the market. Therefore, it is vital to stay informed about regulatory updates.

When designing your labels, aesthetics do matter, but clarity and compliance take precedence. Your label should be legible and durable enough to withstand the conditions your product will go through, whether it's moisture in a bathroom or bright lights at a market stall. Think about using water-resistant labels or packaging that ensures the information stays intact and readable.

The font size is another important consideration. The FDA states that all letters and numbers must be at least 1/16 inch in height based on the lower case letter "o." This ensures that your labels are easily readable. It might be tempting to use artistic, elaborate fonts, but always balance creativity with readability. Be sure to test your labels in various lighting conditions to ensure they're legible from different angles and distances.

Consider the use of additional labeling elements that can enhance the appeal of your products while also providing valuable information. This can include icons, such as "Vegan" or "Cruelty-Free," which quickly communicate the benefits and ethical considerations of your soap. Certifications from recognized bodies can further bolster the authenticity and trustworthiness of your product claims.

Barcodes are another aspect to think about, especially if you plan to sell your soaps in retail stores. A Universal Product Code (UPC) can streamline the process of inventory management for you and your retailers. It's an investment upfront but can significantly ease the operations as you scale up your business.

Eco-friendly labeling is a growing trend. Consider using recycled paper or biodegradable materials for your packaging. Not only does this appeal to environmentally-conscious consumers, but it also aligns with the ethos of creating natural and sustainable products. Paired with a minimalistic design, this approach can create a strong, positive first impression.

Don't forget about the back of the label! This real estate can be utilized to provide additional information that might not fit on the front. You can include usage instructions, storage tips, or a brief story about your soapmaking journey. It's an opportunity to engage with your customers on a more personal level, enriching their experience and creating a connection to your brand.

Remember, compliance doesn't end once your product hits the shelves. Regularly review regulatory guidelines as they can change. Subscribe to industry newsletters, take part in relevant forums, and consider joining a professional body that keeps you abreast of the latest developments. By staying informed, you will not only stay compliant but also ahead of the curve in an ever-evolving market.

Enlisting the help of a legal professional familiar with cosmetic and soap regulations can also be worth the investment. They can review your labels, ensure your compliance with federal and state laws, and help you navigate any legal complexities that may arise.

Finally, be attentive to customer feedback regarding your labels. If customers are frequently asking questions about the ingredients or how to use your soap, it might be a sign that your labels need improvement. Clear, concise, and honest labeling will go a long way in building a loyal customer base and enhancing the credibility of your products.

In summary, effective labeling is more than just a legal obligation; it's a cornerstone of your brand's identity and a key tool for customer engagement. By adhering to regulations and embracing best practices, you lay a solid foundation for trust and reliability, ensuring that your soapmaking journey is as successful as it is sustainable.

Chapter 19: Troubleshooting Common Soapmaking Issues

Even the most experienced soapmakers encounter challenges that can turn a batch of soap from flawless to flawed in seconds. Acceleration and ricing can be particularly frustrating, often caused by additives or temperature fluctuations. If your soap batter thickens too quickly, try mixing your lye solution and oils at a lower temperature and avoiding fragrance oils known to accelerate trace. Soda ash, a chalky layer forming on soap surfaces, can be prevented by covering your soap during the curing process, using distilled water, and ensuring adequate ventilation. Should it still appear, a simple steam treatment or washing the soap surface with a soft cloth can restore its aesthetic. By understanding the root causes and solutions to these common issues, you can refine your soapmaking process and turn every setback into a stepping stone toward success.

Dealing with Acceleration and Ricing

When making soap, two of the most common issues you're likely to encounter are acceleration and ricing. These phenomena can throw even experienced soapmakers for a loop. But don't worry—understanding why they happen and how to manage them can turn these potential pitfalls into manageable bumps on your soapmaking journey. So, let's dive into the intricacies of acceleration and ricing without the usual panic.

First, let's talk about *acceleration*. Acceleration occurs when your soap mixture thickens faster than you had planned. This can be triggered by various factors like temperature, the types of oils and butters used, and, most commonly, the essential oils or fragrances added. It's particularly prevalent in cold process soapmaking. The key to handling acceleration is preparedness and awareness of your ingredients. For instance, spicy or floral essential oils like clove, cinnamon, and lavender are notorious accelerants.

When formulating your recipe, always keep an eye on which oils you're combining. Oils and butters that are solid at room temperature, like coconut oil or shea butter, tend to speed up trace. Balancing these with slower-tracing oils such as olive oil or sunflower oil can help mitigate acceleration. Planning your design accordingly also helps. If you know you're working with quick-tracing ingredients, opt for simpler designs or techniques that don't require a long working time. Have everything prepped and within arm's reach before you start—this way, if your soap does accelerate, you can still pour and mold it with minimal fuss.

On to *ricing*. This odd-sounding problem happens when your soap mixture looks like it has grains of rice floating in it. Ricing usually occurs upon the addition of certain fragrance or essential oils that cause the soap mixture to separate or seize. It doesn't make for a pleasant sight, but it's not the end of the world. The solution to this problem often lies in warming up your oils and lye solution, ensuring they are within a similar temperature range before mixing them together.

Another preventive measure for ricing is to carefully check the compatibility of your fragrance or essential oils. Not all essential oils are soap-friendly, and some commercial fragrances contain additives that can destabilize the soap mixture. Doing a small patch test by blending a tiny amount of the chosen fragrance or essential oil with a bit of your prepared soap batter can save you from a large-scale ricing disaster.

Even experienced soapmakers can't always predict when acceleration or ricing will occur, so having a Plan B is a good practice. If you find your soap batter accelerating or ricing during mixing, you can opt for the hot process method, which involves cooking the soap mixture. The heat can help melt and blend the mixture smoothly back together, effectively saving your batch. Though it might alter the texture and appearance, you still end up with a usable, skin-friendly soap.

Moreover, adjusting your mixing technique can offer a big relief. Instead of stick blending continuously, use short bursts of blending intermixed with hand stirring. This can slow down the pace at which your soap thickens, giving you more working time. Also, starting with your oils and lye at lower temperatures (around 90°F to 110°F) can slow down saponification, providing more time to work with the soap before it hardens up.

Sudden acceleration and ricing can feel frustrating, especially when you've planned a beautiful design. But every soapmaker faces these challenges at some point. Each instance is an opportunity to learn and refine your process. Keeping a detailed soap journal can be incredibly useful. Documenting the types and amounts of oils, butters, essential oils, and fragrances used—along with temperatures and any notable observations—will help identify patterns and potential triggers for these issues.

Importantly, don't be afraid to embrace imperfection. Some of the most unique and interesting soaps come from batches that didn't go exactly as planned. Acceleration and ricing might change your original design, but they can lead to beautiful, rustic, and often surprising results that customers and gift recipients find charming and unique.

Ultimately, the more you familiarize yourself with your ingredients and how they interact, the better equipped you'll be to handle acceleration and ricing. While these challenges might initially seem like setbacks, they're part of the intricate dance that makes soapmaking an ever-evolving craft. Embrace the journey, keep experimenting, and you'll continue to grow both in skill and creativity.

By understanding the causes and solutions to acceleration and ricing, you'll add valuable troubleshooting skills to your soapmaking toolkit. With these skills in hand, you can transform potential soapmaking catastrophes into opportunities for new techniques and designs, pushing the boundaries of what's possible in your soapy creations.

Preventing and Fixing Soda Ash

Soda ash is a common but often frustrating occurrence in cold process soapmaking. This whitish powder can form on the surface of your soap, leaving it looking less than perfect. While it doesn't affect the soap's usability, it can be aesthetically unappealing, especially if you're aiming for smooth, vibrant bars. Understanding why soda ash forms and how to prevent it is crucial for any soapmaker aiming for professional-looking results.

Soda ash forms due to a reaction between the lye water and carbon dioxide in the air. This often happens when the soap is still in its initial curing stages. You'll typically notice soda ash appearing within the first 24 to 48 hours after pouring your soap into molds. An important factor that accelerates the formation of soda ash is the high pH level in newly made soap.

So, how do you prevent this from happening in the first place? One effective method is to control your workspace environment. Ensure that your soap molds are covered immediately after pouring to minimize exposure to air. This can be accomplished by using plastic wrap, wax paper, or the lid of the mold itself. Sealing the molds helps reduce air exposure, limiting the formation of soda ash on the soap surface.

Another useful tactic is to spritz the top of your freshly poured soap with isopropyl alcohol. Use a spray bottle to evenly mist the surface. The alcohol forms a barrier that can lessen soda ash formation. Most soapmakers prefer using 91% isopropyl alcohol for this purpose, but 70% can work in a pinch. Be generous but not excessive; a light, even spritz should do the trick.

It's also wise to assess recipe factors. Soaps with higher water content are more susceptible to soda ash. Consider reducing the water amount slightly, but be cautious. Lower water content can hasten trace and make the soap harder to pour and pattern. A standard water reduction by about 10% can often provide a good balance, but this varies per recipe. Experimenting and taking detailed notes will help you understand what's best for your specific soap batch.

Temperature control plays a significant role too. Higher pouring temperatures can lessen the probability of soda ash forming. Pouring the soap mixture into molds at around 100°F to 110°F ensures a smoother finish. However, if your formulation contains delicate essential oils or botanical additives, take care they don't degrade at higher temperatures.

If soda ash forms despite your best efforts, don't despair; it can be fixed! One of the simplest remedies is to rinse the soap bars under running water and gently wipe the surface using a cloth or sponge. This method often works well, especially if the ash layer is thin. However, be cautious to avoid excessive water exposure which might soften the soap excessively.

Alternatively, you can steam the soap to eliminate soda ash. This method can be particularly effective for larger batches. Simply hold the soap bars over a pot of boiling water (carefully, using tongs or a steaming rack) or use a handheld garment steamer. The steam will dissolve the soda ash, leaving a smooth and clean surface behind. Just ensure the bars are cooled and dried thoroughly before wrapping or packaging them.

Another artistic trick is to incorporate texturing and decorative elements into your soap design deliberately. Using botanicals, textured molds, or embedding elements can divert attention away from any soda ash that does occur. This not only camouflages minor imperfections but also adds a unique touch to each bar, making them truly one of a kind.

Finally, if soda ash remains persistent despite these efforts, you might consider embracing it as a natural part of your soap's aesthetic. While not traditional, some soap makers find beauty in the soft, frosted appearance that soda ash provides. This viewpoint encourages acceptance and creativity, allowing for a more organic, rustic charm in your handmade soaps.

Preventing and fixing soda ash may require some adjustments in your soapmaking process, but the reward is beautifully finished bars that reflect your care and craftsmanship. Keep experimenting with different techniques to understand what works best for you. This journey toward mastery isn't just about preventing problems but also about refining your skills and embracing the learning curve. Happy soapmaking!

Chapter 20:
Advanced Soapmaking Designs

Unleashing your creativity with advanced soapmaking designs can transform your handmade soaps into works of art and elevate your craft to the next level. Embrace embedding and layering techniques to create stunning, multi-dimensional bars that captivate and intrigue. Master the in-the-pot swirl to achieve mesmerizing patterns that leave a lasting impression. Use a variety of molds, from intricate silicone shapes to custom wooden frames, to give your soaps unique forms and textures. Never underestimate the power of experimentation; combining vibrant natural colorants and botanicals can yield unexpected, delightful results. With practice and a daring spirit, your soap designs can become an expression of your artistry, setting your products apart in any market, and inspiring others in the soapmaking community.

Embedding and Layering Techniques

Embedding and Layering are advanced methods used to create visually stunning and unique soaps. These techniques are a step beyond basic soapmaking and involve a combination of artistry and technical skill. By incorporating embedding and layering, you can produce soaps with intricate designs, varied colors, and complex patterns that not only look beautiful but also provide different textures and sensory experiences for the user. If you're ready to take your soapmaking to the next level, these methods are an excellent way to showcase your creativity and craftsmanship.

Let's start with *embedding*. This technique involves placing pre-made soap pieces or other materials into your freshly poured soap base. The embedded items can be anything from small soap shapes, botanicals, or even toys, as long as they are safe and non-toxic. To ensure a successful embed, you need to think about the placement, the type of soap base you'll use to hold the embed in place, and how the embed will interact with the other ingredients. Typically, melt and pour soap bases are ideal for embedding because they allow for precise placement and setting.

When embedding, it's crucial that the temperature of the soap base is just right. If the base is too hot, it might melt or distort your embed. Conversely, if the base is too cool, the embed might not adhere properly. Aim for a "Goldilocks" zone where the base is warm enough to mold around the embed without compromising its shape. This temperature management ensures that all elements fuse seamlessly, producing a cohesive and visually appealing bar of soap.

A helpful tip for embedding is to use alcohol spray. Spritzing both the embed and the melt and pour soap base with alcohol helps eliminate bubbles and creates a better bond between the layers. This is particularly useful when embedding small, intricate shapes that may trap air. The alcohol evaporates, leaving a smooth, bubble-free surface, giving your soap a polished look.

Now, let's shift our focus to *layering* techniques. Layering involves pouring multiple layers of soap, each with distinct colors, scents, or textures, into the same mold. The key to successful layering is timing and consistency. Each layer must be firm enough to support the next but not so hard that they don't bond together. Patience is essential, as well as a well-thought-out plan for the sequence of your layers.

One popular method for creating layers is the use of dividers. Dividers can be inserted into your mold to section off areas for different layers. Once the soap has started to set, the dividers can be carefully removed, leaving clean, straight lines. This approach allows for a high level of precision and creative control, enabling you to produce striking, geometric designs.

Layering offers the opportunity to experiment with various textures by incorporating different additives in each layer. For example, you can have a smooth, opaque bottom layer followed by a textured layer with exfoliants such as oatmeal or seeds, and then topped with a transparent layer containing delicate botanicals. By playing with texture, you not only create a visual contrast but also enhance the functional properties of your soap.

Color is another critical element of layering. The sky's the limit when it comes to choosing colors, but it's essential to consider how they will look together. Harmonious color palettes can create a soothing and cohesive design, while contrasting colors can make your layers pop. Micas, natural clays, and plant-based colorants are excellent options for achieving vibrant, stable colors in your layers.

To prevent the layers from bleeding into each other, ensure that each layer is adequately set before pouring the next one. This can take some trial and error, especially when working with cold process soap that continues to saponify and change consistency as it cures. A good practice is to wait until the previous layer forms a thick "trace," where it is firm enough to support the next layer but still soft enough to bond well.

A fascinating variation of layering is the *gradient layer*. This technique involves gradually changing colors or shades between layers, creating a beautiful ombre or gradient effect. To achieve this look, start with your base layer color and make slight adjustments to the colorants for each subsequent layer. This subtle transition from one color to the next can produce a mesmerizing and professional-looking soap.

Another exciting approach is the *spoon swirling technique*. While this can be part of layering, it adds an element of fluid artistry. After pouring two or more layers, you use a spoon or a tool to gently swirl the soap in a figure-eight motion. This creates intricate swirls and patterns that are unique to each bar. The trick is to swirl just enough to blend the layers without over-mixing, maintaining the integrity of each color.

Safety should always be at the forefront of your mind, especially when experimenting with advanced techniques like embedding and layering. When working with melt and pour bases, always monitor the temperature to avoid burns. For cold process soap, remember to wear gloves, goggles, and long sleeves to protect yourself from lye, which can cause skin irritation or burns if it comes into contact with your skin.

Layering and embedding are transformative techniques in soapmaking that open up a world of creative possibilities. They challenge you to refine your skills, think beyond the basics, and push the boundaries of what handmade soap can be. Whether you're creating a multi-layered masterpiece or embedding whimsical shapes, these methods allow you to infuse artistry into each bar, making your creations not just soap, but a reflection of your passion and innovation.

For those ready to elevate their soapmaking journey, practice and experimentation are key. Don't be afraid to try new combinations, tweak your recipes, and even make mistakes. Each attempt brings you closer to mastering these techniques and finding your unique style. Imagine the delight on a friend's face when they unwrap a soap that looks like it belongs in a high-end boutique, crafted with your own hands and creativity.

The beauty of embedding and layering lies in their ability to transform a simple bar of soap into an experience. With each use, the layers reveal more of their intricate design, and the embedded elements slowly emerge, surprising and delightful. These techniques not only enhance the aesthetic appeal but also the emotional connection to the craftsman, making every wash a reminder of the artistry and care poured into its creation.

Embrace the challenge of embedding and layering techniques to advance your soapmaking craft. With each bar you produce, you'll gain new insights, refine your methods, and most importantly, showcase your creativity and dedication to natural, handmade products. Dive into the world of advanced soap design, and let your imagination guide your hands.

Mastering the In-The-Pot Swirl

In-The-Pot Swirl is a fascinating technique in soapmaking that combines art with science, creating mesmerizing patterns that can take your handcrafted soap to the next level. This method allows for the blending of different colored soap batters in a single pot, resulting in unique, marble-like designs once the soap is sliced. It's a technique that might seem daunting at first, but with a bit of practice and a dash of creativity, you'll soon be transforming ordinary soap into extraordinary works of art.

The first step in mastering the in-the-pot swirl is preparation. Before you even think about swirling, you need to make sure that your soap base is ready and that all your colors are prepped. Choose your design colors carefully; complementary colors work well together and can create a striking visual effect. The soap batter should be at a thin to medium trace, as this will give you enough fluidity to swirl effectively without losing the definition of the swirls. Prepare your colorants by mixing them with a small portion of your soap batter until they achieve a smooth consistency.

Next, it's time to combine your colors. Pour one of your colored soap batters into the pot containing the base soap batter. Add the additional colors in different sections of the pot, being mindful not to over-mix at this stage. You'll typically want to pour from a certain height, like six inches above the base, to ensure the colors penetrate deeper into the base batter. Watch as they create their own initial patterns—it's like watching a mini art show right in your pot.

Once all your colors are in the pot, it's swirling time! This part requires a gentle touch. Using a spatula or a wooden stick, give the batter 1-2 gentle stirs in one direction, then another 1-2 stirs in the opposite direction. The goal here isn't to mix the colors completely but to create beautiful, intricate swirls that are apparent when you cut the soap. You'll develop a feel for how much swirling to do with practice; too much can muddy the colors, while too little might not give you the defined swirls you desire.

Pours and molds play an essential role in this process. Once you're satisfied with your swirl, carefully pour or spoon the batter into your soap mold. Pour along the length of the mold and at varying heights to further distribute the colors and create additional marbling effects. This is where the final magic happens. Each pour will create a different effect, so experiment with different pouring techniques to see what works best for you.

An often-overlooked aspect of the in-the-pot swirl is temperature. The temperature of your soap batter can significantly impact the result. Working at lower temperatures can give you more time to swirl, as the batter takes longer to thicken. On the other hand, slightly warmer batters might create more fluid swirls but require quicker work. It's all about finding that sweet spot that works best for your particular recipe and chosen colors.

Let's not forget about the impact of fragrances and essential oils. Some essential oils accelerate trace, meaning your batter can thicken quickly, limiting your swirling time. Be aware of how your chosen scents interact with soap batter. If you're working with a rapid-tracing essential oil, you might want to mix it into the base before adding your colors to ensure you have maximum time to achieve those perfect swirls.

One thing you'll quickly appreciate about in-the-pot swirling is that no two soaps will ever be identical. This single technique can offer endless variation and creativity, from simple two-color swirls to complex multi-hued designs. Keeping a soapmaking journal can be extremely valuable here. Document your recipes, color choices, swirling motions, and outcomes. Over time, this will become an invaluable resource, helping you to refine your skills and replicate particularly successful patterns.

In the world of soapmaking, patience and experimentation go hand-in-hand. Don't be disheartened if your first few attempts don't turn out as expected. Every misstep is a learning opportunity and will bring you closer to mastering the in-the-pot swirl. Watch your soap closely as it saponifies and sets; sometimes, patterns evolve as the soap hardens, revealing beautiful swirls you didn't initially notice.

As you build confidence, start pushing the boundaries. Try incorporating clays, micas, or natural colorants to see how they interact within the in-the-pot swirl technique. Each of these additives will bring its own twist to your designs, opening up new possibilities for creativity and uniqueness in your soap bars.

Finally, remember that the in-the-pot swirl isn't just about visual appeal. It's about the entire sensory experience. Think about how the colors, fragrances, and textures work together to create a soap that's not only beautiful but also luxurious to use. From the moment someone picks up your handcrafted bar, they should feel the passion and technique that went into making it.

Mastering the in-the-pot swirl is a journey—a blend of science, art, and a touch of alchemy. With each batch, you'll discover new nuances and techniques that can be applied to improve both the aesthetic and functional qualities of your soap. Embrace the process, enjoy the experimentation, and welcome the unexpected results along the way. The beauty of handcrafted soap lies in its uniqueness, and with the in-the-pot swirl, your creations are bound to stand out as uniquely yours.

Chapter 21:
Scaling Up: Tips for Larger Batches

Scaling up your soapmaking process for larger batches can feel like a natural progression once you've mastered the basics and are ready to take your craft or business to the next level. It's crucial to ensure consistency and quality, safeguarding the integrity of each bar, whether you're making tens or hundreds at a time. Begin by upgrading your equipment to handle bigger volumes efficiently—larger mixing containers, industrial-sized molds, and precise measuring tools are key. Prioritize meticulous record-keeping to replicate successful batches and troubleshoot any discrepancies. Quality control becomes paramount; regular pH testing, maintaining accurate temperatures, and vigilant monitoring during saponification will help prevent common issues. Additionally, consider implementing systemized workflow practices to streamline production, such as batch numbering and detailed ingredient tracking. With the right preparation and attention to detail, scaling up can be a seamless transition that fosters creativity and growth in your soapmaking journey.

Equipment for Bigger Batches

Once you've mastered the basics of soapmaking, moving to larger batches is the natural next step. Scaling up production brings its own set of challenges and rewards. To maintain consistency and quality while maximizing efficiency, you'll need specialized equipment. Expanding your soapmaking operations not only makes sense if you're thinking of turning your hobby into a small business, but it also allows you to experiment with more complex recipes and techniques.

One of the primary benefits of producing soap in larger quantities is the ability to lower costs on both ingredients and time. However, making bigger batches also means dealing with larger volumes of hot oils and caustic lye, requiring increased attention to safety and accuracy. The first piece of equipment you'll need to consider is a larger scale for weighing ingredients. Precision is crucial when scaling up recipes, and having a reliable, larger-capacity digital scale can make a world of difference.

A commercial-grade stick blender is another essential tool when working on bigger batches. While your trusty handheld model may have been perfect for small amounts, large volumes need a more powerful motor. This will ensure you blend the lye and oils quickly and evenly, preventing issues like false trace. It's worth investing in a high-quality, durable stick blender that can handle the demands of larger batches without overheating.

Mixing vats and larger pots are also necessary for bigger quantities. Stainless steel or heat-resistant plastic containers are recommended, as they are both durable and easy to clean. Look for pots with high sides to minimize splashing and ensure you have enough space to stir your mixture thoroughly. A large stainless steel pot can also double as a melting container for your oils and butters, eliminating the need for multiple pieces of equipment.

When it comes to pouring your larger soap mixtures, having several big molds is indispensable. Silicone molds are ideal because of their flexibility and ease of use. They come in various shapes and sizes, allowing you to create multiple bars at once. Consider also acquiring loaf molds that can batch several pounds of soap per pour. These larger molds will save you time and effort when creating bulk batches.

Curing racks or shelves are vital for those making soap in larger batches. Proper curing is non-negotiable, and providing ample space for your soaps to dry out is crucial. A well-ventilated area with sturdy shelves will allow your soaps to cure uniformly. You might want to invest in wire shelving units that can accommodate a significant number of soap bars without hogging too much space in your workspace.

Temperature control becomes increasingly important as the size of your batches grows. An infrared thermometer can provide quick, accurate readings without coming into contact with your mixture. Keeping your oils and lye solution at the correct temperatures ensures consistent results, minimizing the risk of batch-to-batch variations.

If you're aiming for a truly professional setup, consider incorporating a soap cutter designed for large loaves. These tools can significantly streamline the cutting process, giving you uniformly sized bars with minimal effort. A multi-wire cutter can slice through a large loaf in seconds, saving you considerable time compared to cutting each bar individually with a knife.

Safety should always be a priority, especially when working on a larger scale. Personal protective equipment (PPE) like gloves, goggles, and long sleeves are even more crucial as the potential for spills and splashes increases. Consider setting up an emergency eyewash station and accessible first-aid kit in your soapmaking area. Stainless steel worktables can also be a good investment, providing sturdy, easy-to-clean surfaces for your operations.

Additionally, storage for your ingredients and finished products is vital in a larger-scale soapmaking operation. Invest in airtight containers to keep your oils, butters, and essential oils fresh. Labeling everything clearly can save you a lot of time and confusion down the line. Shelving units or storage cabinets can help keep your workspace organized and accessible, making your entire operation run more smoothly.

Maintaining consistency in each batch becomes more challenging as you scale up. Record-keeping tools like batch logs are invaluable for tracking ingredient amounts, temperatures, and curing times. Software programs designed for small producers can also help manage inventory, formulate recipes, and even handle sales and customer relations if you're selling your handmade soaps.

For those looking to dive completely into professional-grade soapmaking, investing in an automatic soap mixer can drastically change your workflow. These machines are engineered to blend and trace soap mixtures uniformly, taking much of the manual labor out of the equation. While they represent a significant investment, they could be a game-changer for high-volume production.

Another consideration is the inclusion of large-capacity soap dispensers and packaging equipment. These are essential if you plan to sell your soap in significant quantities. Dispensers facilitate the quick and efficient pouring of liquid soap into molds or bottles, ensuring each unit is filled consistently. Packaging equipment, such as heat sealers for shrink wraps, can provide a professional finish to your products, making them market-ready.

In summary, scaling up your soapmaking requires thoughtful investments in equipment designed for larger volumes. From upgraded blenders to massive molds, every piece of gear helps you maintain quality and consistency while increasing your output. The right equipment does more than just handle greater quantities; it enhances your capacity for creativity and innovation. With the right tools, your soapmaking can easily transition from a passionate hobby to a thriving business.

Consistency and Quality Control

These two concepts are the backbone of successful soapmaking, particularly when scaling up production for a business. When you transition from creating small, handcrafted batches to producing larger quantities, maintaining the same high standards becomes both a priority and a challenge. Consistent quality ensures that every bar you produce meets your expectations and satisfies your customers.

To achieve this, it's crucial to develop a standardized process. This involves meticulously documenting every step of your production method. Record the exact measurements of ingredients, temperatures at various stages, and the specific times for mixing and curing. By having this detailed documentation, you can replicate your results time and time again, minimizing the risks of inconsistency.

A reliable quality control system starts with ingredient selection. Ensure that you're sourcing high-quality, consistent raw materials. Essential oils, herbs, and natural colorants can vary from batch to batch, so purchasing from reputable suppliers with stringent quality standards is key. Regularly check the purity and freshness of your materials before incorporating them into your recipes. Inspect for any changes in color, texture, or aroma that might indicate deterioration or contamination.

One way to uphold consistency is by implementing batch testing. This means creating a small sample batch before producing a larger quantity. Evaluate the sample carefully: does it meet the expected texture, scent, and appearance? Conduct stability tests to see how the soap responds over time. This precautionary step can save you from larger scale issues down the line, ensuring that defects are caught early on.

Keeping a clean and organized workspace can't be overstated. Cleanliness directly impacts the quality of your soap. Cross-contamination with other substances can ruin a batch. Regularly sanitize equipment, surfaces, and storage containers to maintain a hygienic environment. This practice not only supports consistent quality but also assures that your workspace meets any regulatory standards that may apply.

Temperature control is another critical factor. Whether you're using the cold process, hot process, or melt and pour methods, monitoring and maintaining the right temperatures for oils, lye solution, and the soap mixture itself is vital. Fluctuations can lead to issues such as separation, uneven texture, and unintended color changes. Invest in high-quality, digital thermometers to get precise readings and maintain consistency.

Mixing techniques also play a significant role in consistency. For larger batches, you might need to upgrade your equipment to industrial mixers that provide uniform blending. Ensure that the mixing time and speed are constant across all batches. If you're hand-stirring, try to replicate the same motions and timing for each production cycle. Even small variations can make a noticeable difference in the final product.

Once the soap is poured into molds, uniformity in cutting and curing is essential. Use consistent mold sizes and shapes to ensure each bar is the same. Automating this process with a professional soap cutter can help achieve precise, even cuts, eliminating human error. Additionally, maintain a consistent environment for curing, with stable humidity and temperature levels. This can be achieved by setting up a dedicated curing room or area with controlled conditions.

Regular evaluation and adjustment are part of maintaining quality control. Gather feedback from your customers and use it constructively to make improvements. Pay attention to recurring compliments and complaints. If a particular batch received high praise for its moisturizing quality or scent longevity, analyze what you did differently and try to replicate that method going forward.

For those managing a growing business, it might be beneficial to invest in lab testing for your soap. This can confirm the pH level, confirm there are no contaminants, and verify that your soaps meet safety standards. While this step involves additional costs, it adds an extra layer of assurance for both you and your customers, building trust in your brand.

The importance of scalability can't be ignored. When scaling up, don't skimp on ingredients or take shortcuts. Instead, ensure that your increases in volume are matched by increases in precision and quality checks. Double-check measurements and possibly employ automated systems to avoid human error. This meticulous attention to detail will help maintain the integrity of your product, even as production increases.

Don't forget about the compliance aspect of a growing soap business. Familiarize yourself with local and international regulations regarding the production and sale of handmade soap. Compliance ensures not only that you're legally protected but also that your customers can trust the safety and effectiveness of your products. Missteps here can be costly, both financially and reputarily.

Documenting customer feedback is another pillar of quality control. Create a system where customers can easily share their experiences with your products, and any issues they might encounter. This direct line of communication can offer invaluable insights into areas needing improvement and aspects you need to maintain or enhance.

Remember, the ultimate goal of consistency and quality control is to create a dependable product that your customers come to love and expect. It's this reliability that will distinguish your soaps from the myriad of options available on the market, embedding a sense of trust and loyalty among your clientele. When every bar produced carries the same level of quality and care, you are not just building a product; you're building a brand that stands for excellence.

Chapter 22: Selling Your Handmade Soaps

Now that you've mastered the art of soapmaking, it's time to turn your passion into a thriving business. First, you must set up your soapmaking business with the right foundation—this involves more than just making great soap. Begin by choosing a business name that reflects your brand's essence and registering it with the necessary local authorities. Next, create an engaging online presence through a well-designed website and active social media profiles. Utilize platforms like Etsy or your e-commerce site to reach a broader audience. Effective marketing is crucial; share your story, offer samples, and engage with your community to build a loyal customer base. Don't forget to follow legal requirements, including labeling regulations and good manufacturing practices. By combining these strategies with your unique creations, you can create a successful soapmaking business that not only brings in revenue but also brings joy to your customers and supports eco-friendly practices.

Setting Up a Soapmaking Business

This can be an incredibly rewarding venture if you possess a genuine passion for crafting natural, enchanting soaps and a keen eye for detail. Transitioning from a hobbyist to a business owner requires thorough planning and dedication, but with the right strategy, it's possible to carve out a profitable niche in the market.

The first step in laying down a strong foundation for your soapmaking business is conducting market research. Take the time to understand the trends, demands, and preferences of your potential customers. Research local and online marketplaces, examine what successful soap brands are offering, and identify gaps that your products can fill. Pay close attention to the types of soaps that are currently trending, such as those that emphasize organic ingredients, have unique aromatherapy benefits, or are eco-friendly.

Next, creating a unique brand identity will be critical. Your brand should reflect your values, target audience, and the unique qualities of your soap products. Start by designing an eye-catching logo, developing a compelling brand story, and creating a palette of consistent branding elements such as fonts, colors, and packaging styles. Your branding will set you apart from competitors and help customers easily recognize and remember your products.

Once your brand identity is established, focus on developing a comprehensive business plan. This plan should outline your business objectives, target market, product line, pricing strategy, and marketing plan. Additionally, it should detail your operational procedures, including sourcing raw materials, production methods, and quality control measures. A well-structured business plan will serve as a roadmap for your business's growth and help attract potential investors or secure financing from banks.

Legal considerations play an essential role in setting up your soapmaking business. Ensure that you comply with local regulations and obtain any necessary licenses or permits. In the U.S., the Food and Drug Administration (FDA) oversees regulations pertaining to cosmetics, including handmade soap. Familiarize yourself with labeling requirements, particularly regarding ingredient disclosure and any claims about the benefits of your soap. Adhering to these regulations will not only keep your business lawful but also build trust with customers.

Next, acquiring the right equipment and workspace is crucial for efficient production. Depending on your production scale, invest in high-quality soap molds, mixing equipment, safety gear, and storage solutions for your raw materials. Designate a dedicated workspace, ensuring it is clean, well-organized, and adheres to any local health and safety guidelines. This space will be the heart of your operation, where creativity and precision meet.

Purchasing ingredients in bulk can significantly reduce costs, but it's important to maintain the quality of your inputs. Establish relationships with reliable suppliers who can provide consistent, high-quality oils, butters, essential oils, and other additives. Many suppliers offer wholesale pricing for larger orders, which can help you maximize your profit margins without compromising on the quality of your final product.

Crafting an effective pricing strategy is another critical aspect of your business. Your pricing should cover the cost of materials, labor, and overhead while providing a reasonable profit margin. Research the prices of similar products in the market and position your pricing competitively. Be transparent about the value your customers receive, such as the use of premium ingredients or bespoke formulations, to justify your pricing.

Marketing your soapmaking business effectively is key to gaining visibility and attracting customers. Develop a multi-channel marketing strategy that includes social media, a professional website, email newsletters, and participation in local craft fairs or farmers' markets. Share engaging content that highlights your production process, the benefits of your natural ingredients, and customer testimonials. Utilizing high-quality photography and video can showcase the appeal of your products and foster a connection with your audience.

Building an online presence is particularly vital in the digital age. Set up an attractive, user-friendly e-commerce website where customers can easily browse your products, read detailed descriptions, and make secure purchases. Consider using platforms like Etsy, Amazon Handmade, or your own website if you're tech-savvy. Optimize your site for search engines (SEO) to enhance visibility and drive organic traffic to your store.

Effective financial management is essential for the sustainability of your business. Keep detailed records of your expenses, sales, and profits to monitor your business's financial health. Use accounting software to streamline this process and consider working with a financial advisor or accountant, especially during tax season. Maintaining financial transparency will help you make informed decisions and plan for the future.

Customer service can make or break your business, so strive to provide an exceptional experience from the moment a customer discovers your brand to after their purchase. Offer clear communication, prompt responses to inquiries, and hassle-free returns or exchanges. Encourage customer feedback and use it to continuously improve your products and services.

Lastly, be prepared for growth. As your business gains traction, you might need to scale up your operations. This could involve hiring additional staff, expanding your workspace, or investing in more advanced equipment. Stay adaptable and willing to evolve your business model as the market and your customer base change.

Embrace the journey of **setting up a soapmaking business** with dedication, creativity, and a commitment to delivering the best products to your customers. Each bar of soap you craft is not only a testament to your skill but also a piece of your brand's story. With careful planning and a passion for excellence, you can transform your passion for soapmaking into a thriving and successful business.

Marketing and Selling Online

Taking your product online can open the doors to a vast audience eager to discover your natural soaps crafted with herbs and essential oils. The digital marketplace allows you to showcase your unique creations to potential customers worldwide, making it an invaluable tool for growing your soapmaking business. Let's dive into some key strategies for establishing and enhancing your online presence, as well as converting casual visitors into loyal customers.

First and foremost, it's essential to create an appealing and functional website. This is your virtual storefront and the first impression for many customers. Invest in a user-friendly platform that allows easy navigation, secure transactions, and responsive design to ensure it looks good on any device. High-quality images and detailed descriptions of your soaps are crucial. They not only showcase the beauty of your products but also inform customers about the ingredients and benefits, emphasizing the natural and eco-friendly aspect that sets your soaps apart.

Consider integrating an e-commerce platform like Shopify or WooCommerce. These platforms simplify the process of listing products, managing inventory, and processing payments, leaving you more time to focus on creating your soaps. Additionally, having a blog on your site where you share soapmaking tips, the benefits of using natural ingredients, and behind-the-scenes content can help build a connection with your audience, establishing you as an authority in the natural soapmaking community.

Social media is another powerful tool for marketing and selling your soaps online. Platforms such as Instagram, Facebook, and Pinterest are particularly effective for showcasing the aesthetic appeal of your products. Post regularly with high-quality photos, engaging captions, and use relevant hashtags to increase your visibility. Stories and live videos can give your audience a peek into your soapmaking process, helping to personalize your brand and build trust with potential customers.

Don't underestimate the power of testimonials and reviews. Positive feedback from satisfied customers can significantly impact purchasing decisions. Encourage your customers to leave reviews on your website and share their experience on social media. Offering a small discount or a free sample of a new product in exchange for a review can be an effective way to generate valuable testimonials.

Email marketing remains one of the most cost-effective methods for reaching your audience. Building an email list allows you to keep in touch with your customers, notifying them of new product launches, special promotions, and exclusive offers. Platforms like Mailchimp and Constant Contact make it easy to design attractive newsletters and manage your subscriber list. Personalize your emails to make your customers feel valued, and consistently provide content that is both informative and engaging.

Search engine optimization (SEO) is another crucial aspect of marketing online. By optimizing your website's content for relevant keywords, you can improve your search engine ranking, making it easier for potential customers to find you. Keywords like "natural soap," "handmade soaps," and "essential oil soap" should be incorporated naturally into your product descriptions, blog posts, and metadata. Tools like Google Analytics can help you understand your site's traffic and identify areas for improvement.

Online marketplaces like Etsy can also be an excellent avenue for selling your soaps. Etsy is known for its community of buyers who value handcrafted and unique items, making it a perfect fit for your natural soaps. Ensure your product listings are optimized with clear titles, detailed descriptions, and professional photos. Participate in Etsy's community forums and network with other sellers to share tips and gain insights into effective selling strategies.

Collaborate with influencers and bloggers who align with your brand's values. These partnerships can introduce your soaps to a wider audience and build credibility. Send samples to influencers who have a following that matches your target market. A well-crafted review or a social media post from a trusted influencer can significantly boost your brand's visibility and credibility.

Remember to track and analyze your marketing efforts. Use analytics tools to monitor website traffic, social media engagement, and email campaign performance. Understanding what's working and what could be improved allows you to refine your strategies and achieve better results over time.

Lastly, consider participating in online events, such as virtual craft fairs and webinars. These events can help you reach new audiences and connect with other soapmakers and enthusiasts. Hosting your own online workshops or tutorials can also position you as an expert in natural soapmaking, attracting customers who are interested in learning more about your process and products.

In conclusion, marketing and selling online require a multifaceted approach. A combination of a strong website, active social media presence, strategic SEO, and engaging email marketing can significantly elevate your business. Remember to stay authentic and true to your brand's values, as this authenticity will resonate with customers and foster loyalty. With persistence and creativity, the digital marketplace can become a thriving platform for your natural soaps.

Chapter 23:
The Future of Soapmaking

The future of soapmaking shines bright with potential and innovation, pushing the boundaries of creativity while embracing sustainability. As more consumers prioritize eco-friendly products, soapmakers are pioneering new techniques to minimize environmental impact, like zero-waste practices and biodegradable packaging. Advances in natural ingredient sourcing ensure ethical harvesting, supporting the global push for responsible consumption. Trends are leaning towards personalized skincare solutions, with makers experimenting with custom blends of herbs, essential oils, and unique additives tailored to individual skin needs. Keeping pulse on cutting-edge research in botanicals and emulsification processes can lead to breakthroughs in texture, longevity, and skin benefits. In this evolving landscape, the fusion of tradition and technology not only enhances the soapmaking craft but also fosters a community committed to ecological stewardship and creative excellence. The journey ahead promises not just cleaner, greener soaps, but a stronger, more informed community of artisans dedicated to nurturing both their craft and the planet.

Trends in Natural Soapmaking

The art of Natural Soapmaking has been evolving rapidly, driven by consumer demands and innovative techniques. More than ever, enthusiasts are looking for ways to make their soaps unique, eco-friendly, and health-conscious. The growing emphasis on sustainability and clean beauty has profoundly influenced the ingredients, processes, and designs in natural soap making. By staying ahead of these trends, whether as a hobbyist or a small business owner, you can create captivating products that resonate with contemporary values.

One of the most notable trends is the increasing use of locally sourced ingredients. Soapmakers are turning to their own backyards—or nearby farms—to find fresh herbs, flowers, and other botanicals. This not only supports local agriculture but also ensures the ingredients are fresh and organically grown. Think of including lavender from your garden for calming soaps or calendula petals for their skin-soothing properties. The farm-to-bar movement echoes the broader farm-to-table trend in the culinary world and adds a unique, personalized touch to your soaps.

Alongside locally sourced ingredients, there's a resurgence in traditional methods and recipes. Many soapmakers are revisiting ancient techniques and incorporating them into modern practices. Cold process and hot process methods, as ancient as they are effective, are being celebrated for their ability to create rich, earthy bars of soap. These traditional methods allow for greater control over ingredient selection and customization, making them a favorite among purists and those interested in heritage crafts.

Natural colorants are also making a big splash. Soapmakers are moving away from synthetic dyes, instead using clays, roots, fruits, and even algae to give their creations vibrant hues. For instance, French green clay and activated charcoal can provide stunning, natural tones without any chemical additives. These colorants not only offer visual appeal but often come with added skincare benefits, enhancing the overall value of the product.

Another exciting trend is the integration of herbal infusions and extracts. By infusing carrier oils with herbs before adding them to the soap mixture, makers can imbue their products with the therapeutic properties of the botanicals. Chamomile-infused oil, for example, can be used in a soap intended to soothe irritated skin. This practice allows for greater creativity and experimentation, leading to products that are both unique and beneficial.

Incorporating exotic and less common oils is gaining traction as well. Oils like argan, kukui nut, and maracuja are becoming popular for their distinctive properties and luxurious feel. These oils often carry a higher price point but can be used as superfatting agents or in specialty lines to justify their inclusion. They're especially appealing to consumers seeking high-end, boutique-style soaps.

A trend worth noting is the rise of zero-waste and eco-friendly packaging. With growing environmental awareness, soapmakers are opting for biodegradable wraps, recycled papers, and compostable labels. Some even go as far as creating 'naked' soaps with no packaging at all, using intricate designs and natural colorants to make the soap itself aesthetically pleasing. This shift not only speaks to sustainability but also appeals to the eco-conscious consumer, aligning with broader movements toward green living.

Technological integration isn't left behind, either. Soapmakers are leveraging social media platforms, online communities, and digital tools to share techniques, sell products, and build brands. Instagram-worthy designs, instructional YouTube videos, and vibrant Pinterest boards have become crucial tools for reaching audiences and showcasing creative prowess. Moreover, online marketplaces and e-commerce platforms enable small-scale artisans to reach a global customer base, breaking down traditional market barriers.

The minimalist approach is another emerging trend, advocating for simple, clean ingredients and straightforward formulations. In this era of heightened ingredient awareness, many consumers prefer soaps made from recognizable components. Labels that list olive oil, coconut oil, and essential oils without a long list of scientific names are comforting to those seeking natural skincare solutions.

The natural soapmaking community isn't just about creating a product; it's about fostering a lifestyle. Workshops, both in-person and virtual, are gaining popularity, offering enthusiasts the opportunity to learn, network, and exchange ideas. These events often include hands-on sessions, expert panels, and collaborative projects, enriching the overall experience. They also reinforce the sense of community and shared passion that is so central to the hobby and profession.

Lastly, inclusivity and customizability are becoming key selling points. Soaps designed for different skin types, ages, and personal preferences ensure that every customer finds something tailored to their needs. This approach can extend to hypoallergenic options, vegan formulations, or even gender-neutral scents. Customization allows small businesses to cater to niche markets, creating a strong, loyal customer base.

Whether you're a seasoned soapmaker or just starting out, staying attuned to these trends can offer a treasure trove of ideas to inspire your next project. The field of natural soapmaking is as dynamic as it is rewarding, with endless possibilities for creative and beneficial products. Embrace these trends, experiment with new techniques, and let your imagination be your guide in crafting soaps that are both beautiful and aligned with contemporary values.

Innovation and Sustainability in the Industry

Sustainability and innovations in soapmaking has become crucial areas of focus in the world of soapmaking, as more enthusiasts and businesses are looking to align their practices with eco-friendly and forward-thinking approaches. With growing awareness about the environmental impact of conventional soap production, soapmakers are striving to incorporate innovative techniques and sustainable materials in their craft. This has resulted in a dynamic shift from traditional methods to more environmentally conscious production processes.

One of the most significant innovations in soapmaking is the use of alternative ingredients that are both sustainable and beneficial to the skin. Traditional soap recipes often rely on palm oil, which has garnered negative attention due to deforestation and habitat destruction linked to palm oil plantations. In response, many soapmakers are turning to palm-free recipes, using alternatives such as olive oil, coconut oil, and shea butter. These ingredients not only offer similar benefits in terms of lather and moisturizing properties but also have a lower environmental footprint.

Another burgeoning trend is the incorporation of locally sourced and organic ingredients. By selecting herbs, essential oils, and other natural additives from local farmers and suppliers, soapmakers are reducing their carbon footprint and supporting their communities. This practice also ensures a higher level of transparency and quality control, as makers can be more confident about the origins and farming practices of their ingredients. It's a beautiful synergy between sustainability and quality that adds immense value to handmade soaps.

Biodegradability is an essential factor in sustainability efforts. Many commercial soaps contain synthetic additives and detergents that do not break down easily, contributing to water pollution. In contrast, handmade natural soaps typically comprise biodegradable ingredients, ensuring that they decompose without harming the environment. This shift is part of a larger movement towards creating products that are not only good for the body but also gentle on the earth.

Packaging innovation is another frontier in sustainable soapmaking. The use of plastic-free, recyclable, and compostable packaging options has grown significantly. Creative packaging solutions such as wrapping soaps in cloth, using plantable seed paper, or opting for recycled cardboard boxes not only minimize waste but often enhance the aesthetic and perceived value of the product. Small tweaks in packaging approach can lead to substantial reductions in environmental impact, and they resonate well with eco-conscious consumers.

The introduction of zero-waste production techniques has also marked a revolutionary step in the industry. This includes rethinking production processes to minimize waste at every stage, from ingredient sourcing to the final product. For instance, soap scraps and leftover materials can be repurposed into new batches, minimizing waste and maximizing resources. Moreover, some soapmakers have adopted techniques that require less water and energy, further reducing their environmental footprint.

Recycling and upcycling are gaining ground as well. Many soapmakers have started to collect used soap pieces from customers to create new bars. This practice not only encourages consumers to return old soap pieces but also fosters a circular economy approach, where products are continually repurposed rather than disposed of. Additionally, repurposing materials such as using old cooking oil from restaurants to make soaps has opened new avenues for reducing waste and promoting sustainability.

Advancements in technology have enabled soapmakers to experiment with innovative formulations and techniques that were previously challenging. High-tech equipment like soap cutters, molds, and temperature-controlled environments allow for precision and consistency in production while reducing manual labor and energy consumption. The use of digital platforms for recipe formulation and testing has also streamlined the process, making it easier to experiment with sustainable ingredients and techniques.

Education and awareness play a pivotal role in driving these innovations forward. Workshops, online courses, and community events dedicated to sustainable soapmaking are spreading valuable knowledge and skills among enthusiasts and professionals alike. As more people gain access to these resources, the movement towards eco-friendly and innovative soapmaking will continue to grow. This sharing of knowledge fosters a community spirit and encourages collective efforts towards a more sustainable future.

Collaborations between soapmakers and other industries have resulted in exciting product developments. For instance, partnerships with the agricultural sector have led to the adoption of farm-based materials, such as goat milk and honey, which not only support local farmers but also enhance the nutritional value of the soap. Moreover, working with environmental organizations has helped soapmakers align their practices with broader sustainability goals, such as reducing plastic waste and protecting natural habitats.

Sustainability and innovation in soapmaking also translate into more transparent and ethical business practices. Consumers today are increasingly discerning and demand more information about the products they purchase. By being transparent about their sourcing methods, production techniques, and sustainability efforts, soapmakers can build a loyal customer base that values ethical consumption. This transparency not only boosts consumer trust but also sets a standard for the industry.

Looking ahead, it's clear that sustainability will continue to be a driving force in soapmaking innovation. As the industry evolves, there will be more emphasis on research and development of new materials that are both skin-friendly and environmentally sustainable. Ingenious solutions for reducing energy consumption, waste material, and water usage will be pivotal in shaping the future landscape of soapmaking.

These efforts will likely lead to breakthroughs that make sustainable soap production more accessible and cost-effective.

Furthermore, the role of technology in propelling the industry towards greater sustainability cannot be understated. Advances in biotechnology, for example, are paving the way for the creation of plant-based alternatives to traditional animal-derived ingredients. Similarly, innovations in renewable energy could potentially power soapmaking operations, reducing their carbon footprint. As these technologies become more mainstream, they will empower soapmakers to create products that are not just beautiful and effective, but also environmentally responsible.

The journey towards sustainable and innovative soapmaking is a continuous one. It involves ongoing learning, experimentation, and adaptation. Each step taken towards a more sustainable practice not only benefits the environment but also inspires others in the industry to follow suit. By embracing these changes, soapmakers can contribute to a larger movement towards environmental stewardship, creating a lasting impact that extends beyond their individual creations.

In conclusion, the soapmaking industry is at a pivotal point where innovation and sustainability are not just trends but essential components of its evolution. By adopting sustainable practices and embracing innovative techniques, soapmakers can create products that are not only superior in quality but also kind to the planet. This alignment of creativity with sustainability promises a bright and responsible future for the art of soapmaking, ensuring that this beloved craft continues to thrive in harmony with our environment.

Chapter 24:
Joining the Soapmaking Community

Becoming an active part of the soapmaking community can significantly enrich your craft and provide you with invaluable support and inspiration. There are numerous forums, workshops, and events that cater to soapmakers of all levels, offering opportunities to share knowledge, troubleshoot issues, and discover new techniques. Engaging with fellow enthusiasts often leads to collaborations and networking that can take your soapmaking to new heights, whether you hobbyist or a small business owner. By immersing yourself in this vibrant community, you not only enhance your skills but also contribute to the collective growth and sustainability of the craft. Reach out, connect, and be open to learning from others' experiences; the relationships you build and the knowledge you gain will be instrumental in your soapmaking journey.

Forums, Workshops, and Events

These community activities are remarkable for bringing soapmaking enthusiasts together, fostering a sense of community and shared passion. Whether you're a seasoned soapmaker or just getting started, these platforms provide invaluable opportunities to connect, learn, and grow. One of the best aspects of engaging in forums is the wealth of knowledge that flows freely among participants. You'll find forums dedicated specifically to natural soapmaking, where experienced crafters share their wisdom, troubleshoot issues, and offer tips on everything from sourcing ingredients to mastering tricky techniques.

Forums often feature dedicated sections for different soapmaking methods, such as cold process, hot process, and melt and pour. Within these categories, you can dive deep into specialized topics like superfatting, saponification values, and the use of essential oils and botanicals. The beauty of these online communities lies in their collaborative spirit; many soapmakers are eager to help others avoid common pitfalls and achieve their creative visions. It's not unusual to find detailed tutorials, step-by-step guides, and even video demonstrations that can demystify complex procedures.

Apart from forums, attending workshops offers a more hands-on approach to learning and connecting with other soapmakers. Workshops can vary widely in scope and scale, ranging from local meet-ups to larger, more structured events hosted by seasoned professionals. Whether you choose an intimate, in-person gathering or a comprehensive virtual seminar, workshops provide a structured environment where you can build your skills and network with like-minded individuals. Many workshops offer the chance to work with unique ingredients and tools that might not be readily accessible, giving you the opportunity to experiment and expand your soapmaking repertoire.

In addition to technique-based workshops, you may also find events focused on specific themes or trends in the soapmaking world. These can include sessions on seasonal soapmaking, eco-friendly practices, or advanced design techniques like embedding and layering. Guest instructors, often experts in the field, bring a unique perspective and can offer insights drawn from their professional experience. These events serve as a melting pot of inspiration, where new ideas and collaborations are born.

Furthermore, workshops are often designed to appeal to a wide range of skill levels, making them accessible to beginners while still offering valuable takeaways for more experienced artisans. For newcomers, there's the benefit of hands-on guidance and the reassurance that comes from learning in a supportive environment. For seasoned soapmakers, advanced workshops offer the chance to refine techniques, explore new materials, and stay updated on industry trends. Workshop facilitators often encourage participants to ask questions and engage in discussions, fostering a collaborative learning experience that benefits everyone involved.

Then there are the larger-scale soapmaking events—conventions, expos, and trade shows—which offer a treasure trove of networking opportunities and industry insights. These events often draw attendees from across the globe, including soapmakers, suppliers, and industry experts. With a packed agenda of seminars, demonstrations, and vendor booths, attendees can immerse themselves in the latest innovations and trends. These events also provide a platform for businesses to showcase their products, making it easier for you to discover new ingredients, tools, and packaging solutions that can elevate your soapmaking practice.

One of the greatest advantages of attending these large events is the opportunity for face-to-face interaction with other soapmakers and industry professionals. In-person connections can lead to collaborations, mentorships, and enduring friendships. Networking with others who share your passion for natural soapmaking can be incredibly motivating and can propel you toward achieving your personal and business goals. Some events even feature networking receptions or round-table discussions, where you can exchange ideas and insights in a more relaxed setting.

To make the most out of these events, consider preparing in advance. Plan which workshops, seminars, or demonstrations you want to attend, and make a list of vendors you want to visit. If you're attending a large convention or expo, it's helpful to review the event schedule and map in advance so you can prioritize your time effectively. Most events also offer opportunities for one-on-one consultations or portfolio reviews, so bringing samples of your work could add another layer of valuable feedback to your experience.

Another great aspect of forums, workshops, and events is their role in fostering a continuous learning journey. Soapmaking, like any craft, involves ongoing education and adaptation. Through these platforms, you can keep abreast of the latest techniques, materials, and industry standards. Many forums and event organizers also offer newsletters and online resources, extending the learning experience beyond the scope of the event itself. This continuous engagement ensures that you're always growing, evolving, and staying inspired in your soapmaking journey.

Moreover, these communities often highlight emerging sustainability practices and innovations in the natural soapmaking industry. For soapmakers dedicated to eco-friendly and sustainable methods, this shared commitment can be profoundly motivating. Learning about new ways to reduce waste, source sustainable ingredients, and create environmentally-friendly packaging not only benefits your craft but also helps in promoting a more sustainable world. You might even discover green business practices that can differentiate your products in a competitive market.

So, whether you're engaging with fellow soapmakers in an online forum, attending a local workshop, or participating in a large industry event, the connections you make and the knowledge you gain can profoundly impact your soapmaking journey. These experiences provide a blend of inspiration, education, and community that is hard to replicate on your own. By investing your time and energy into these communal platforms, you're not just enhancing your skills but also enriching your overall experience in the world of natural soapmaking.

Finally, don't hesitate to share your experiences and newfound knowledge with the community. Whether it's a tip you picked up at a workshop or a new technique you learned at an expo, your contributions can help others on their soapmaking journey. The soapmaking community thrives on this spirit of sharing and collaboration, making it a continually evolving and enriching space for everyone involved.

Collaborations and Networking

Finding ways to collaborate and network can be the secret sauce that elevates your soapmaking journey from a solo hobby to a dynamic, thriving venture. In a world where social connections and community support are more accessible than ever, tapping into these networks can offer you a wealth of knowledge, inspiration, and opportunities. There's a palpable excitement in sharing your creations, learning from others, and collectively pushing the boundaries of what's possible.

Imagine for a moment the power of attending a local farmers' market and chatting with fellow soapmakers. These interactions can be more valuable than you might think. They offer a chance to share techniques, suppliers, and experiences that you wouldn't come across sitting alone in your workspace. The act of collaboration fosters a sense of camaraderie and can lead to joint ventures that are mutually beneficial.

One effective way to start networking is by joining online forums and social media groups dedicated to soapmaking. These platforms teem with passionate individuals who are eager to share their expertise. You'll find everything from troubleshooting advice to advanced techniques that you can incorporate into your own process. Think of it as having a virtual soapmaking family that's always ready to lend a hand or offer encouragement.

Moreover, don't underestimate the power of workshops and classes. Attending a soapmaking workshop offers hands-on experience that can be more informative than reading a dozen books. Here, you can meet experienced soapmakers, ask specific questions, and observe techniques up close. Plus, these events often include networking opportunities where you can connect with folks who share your passion.

Harnessing the potential of online platforms extends beyond forums. Instagram, Pinterest, and YouTube are treasure troves of inspiration and instructional content. By following influential soapmakers, you can gain insights into trends, learn new techniques, and discover innovative design ideas. Collaborating with these influencers through shout-outs or co-created content can also boost your own visibility.

Networking isn't just about gaining knowledge; it's also about sharing. Teach what you know, share your failures and triumphs, and be generous with your wisdom. The more you give, the more you get back in return. This reciprocal exchange strengthens the community and paves the way for future collaborations.

In the realm of physical collaborations, consider partnering with other artisans, like candlemakers, essential oil suppliers, or herbalists. Such partnerships can lead to the creation of unique product lines that appeal to a broader audience. Imagine a themed gift basket featuring your soap and complementary products from your collaborators. This approach not only amplifies your reach but also adds a layer of novelty that customers love.

Local community events and fairs are also excellent venues for networking and collaboration. Participating in these events allows you to meet potential customers face-to-face and build lasting relationships. These interactions provide immediate feedback and help you understand your market better. Sometimes, the most rewarding collaborations stem from a casual conversation at a local fair.

Another avenue to explore is trade associations or guilds. Being part of a professional organization lends credibility and opens doors to a plethora of resources. These bodies often provide industry-specific training, marketing opportunities, and platforms for showcasing your work. It's also a great way to stay updated on industry standards and best practices.

For those with a more entrepreneurial spirit, collaborative projects can scale your business in innovative ways. Group buy initiatives, where multiple soapmakers pool resources to purchase raw materials in bulk, can significantly lower costs. Additionally, joint marketing efforts or co-hosted events can draw larger crowds and create more buzz than single-handed efforts.

Lastly, don't forget to leverage digital tools that facilitate collaboration. Project management apps, video conferencing, and cloud-based file sharing can make working with others a seamless experience, no matter the physical distance. Technology has essentially erased geographical barriers, making global collaboration a feasible and often enriching prospect.

Incorporating collaborations and networking into your soapmaking practice isn't just beneficial; it can be transformative. The collective creativity and shared resources you gain from these interactions are invaluable. Embrace these opportunities, and you'll find not just growth in your skills and business, but lasting friendships and an enriched experience. The soapmaking community is vibrant and welcoming—don't hesitate to dive in and make the most of it.

Chapter 25:
Continuing Your Soapmaking Journey

As you move forward in your soapmaking journey, remember that the learning never truly ends—there's always something new and exciting to discover. Dive into further educational resources, whether through advanced workshops, online courses, or well-reviewed literature, to continually enhance your skills and knowledge. Embrace experimentation with novel ingredients, unique designs, and innovative techniques to keep your creative juices flowing and stay ahead of the trends. Your growth as a soapmaker comes from both your successes and your challenges, so don't be afraid to push beyond your comfort zone. By staying curious and dedicated, you'll not only perfect your craft but also inspire others in the soapmaking community. Here's to a future filled with bubbles, creativity, and sustainable practices that bring joy and beauty into the world.

Further Education and Resources

These play an essential role in advancing your skills and knowledge in soapmaking. Whether you're a novice just starting out or an experienced artisan looking to refine your craft, the journey doesn't have to end with the pages of this book. Delving deeper into the world of natural soapmaking can open up new avenues of creativity, sustainability, and even potential business opportunities.

Start by exploring advanced courses offered by reputable institutions and websites dedicated to soapmaking. Online platforms such as Udemy, Coursera, and professional soapmaking schools provide a wealth of structured courses that cover advanced techniques, scientific formulations, and even business management tips for those looking to commercialize their products. Reading reviews and getting recommendations from the soapmaking community can go a long way in selecting quality courses that fit your learning style and goals.

Don't overlook the vast array of literature available on the subject. Books written by seasoned soapmakers offer deeper insights and often include recipes, tips, and troubleshooting advice that can be invaluable. Some notable mentions include works by experts who have been pioneers in the field, just as you encountered in this book. These texts serve as reference guides you can revisit, offering inspiration and solutions when you hit a creative or technical snag.

Attending workshops and conferences is another excellent way to continue your education. Engaging in hands-on workshops allows you to experience new techniques firsthand. You'll also have the opportunity to ask questions and get immediate feedback. Conferences, on the other hand, are a fantastic way to stay current with industry trends, network with fellow soapmakers, and even meet suppliers and distributors if you're thinking about scaling up your production.

Don't underestimate the power of joining online forums and social media groups dedicated to soapmaking. Communities on platforms like Facebook, Reddit, and specialized forums provide a collaborative environment where members share experiences, pose questions, and offer advice. The sense of camaraderie and support in these groups can be both motivational and educational. You'll find that being part of such communities not only helps in solving immediate issues but also keeps you inspired with new ideas and trends in the soapmaking world.

If you're looking into specialized areas such as herbal infusions or advanced essential oil blending, consider more focused courses and resources. Aromatherapy schools and herbalism courses often delve deeply into topics that are only briefly covered here. Mastering these subjects can enhance the therapeutic qualities of your soaps and expand your product offerings.

Research and experimentation are key components of continuous learning. Don't be afraid to experiment with new ingredients, techniques, and styles in your soapmaking process. Keep detailed notes on your successes and failures to build a personalized knowledge base. Over time, this documentation will become an invaluable resource, guiding you to perfect your recipes and innovate your product line.

Documentaries and instructional videos can also be incredibly helpful. Visual learners may find that watching experienced soapmakers in action helps demystify complex techniques. Platforms like YouTube host a plethora of channels dedicated to soapmaking, each offering tutorials, product reviews, and detailed guides. Select channels with good reputations and high-quality content to ensure you're getting accurate and valuable information.

Collaborating with others can also be a powerful way to expand your knowledge. Partner with other soapmakers for joint projects or exchange knowledge with crafters skilled in different areas such as candle making, lotion crafting, or even perfumery. This exchange of ideas could lead to unique product innovations and learning opportunities.

Stay updated with current research and developments in the field of natural products and sustainability. Scientific journals and publications often carry studies on the properties of various natural ingredients, innovations in eco-friendly packaging, and advancements in green chemistry, which can all be leveraged to enhance your soapmaking practice.

For those considering the business side of soapmaking, knowledge in entrepreneurial skills is crucial. Business courses, either general or those specifically tailored to soapmaking and natural products, can guide you through the aspects of marketing, sales strategies, financial management, and legal regulations. This holistic approach ensures that you not only create high-quality products but also run a successful business.

Lastly, never underestimate the inspiration derived from simply perusing nature itself. Walks in botanical gardens, visits to herb farms, and even casual strolls in a park can spark creativity. Pay close attention to the textures, colors, and fragrances of plants and flowers. You might discover new ingredients to experiment with or even new aesthetic designs for your soaps.

As you navigate through these further educational avenues and resources, remember that soapmaking is both an art and a science. Continuous learning, curiosity, and a willingness to experiment will push the boundaries of what you can create. This journey is not just about making soap; it's about embracing a sustainable, creative lifestyle that brings joy and value to both the creator and the user.

Experimentation and Ongoing Learning

Ongoing Learning and experimentation is the heartbeat of the soapmaking craft, an endless journey of discovery where every batch presents new opportunities to refine your skills and expand your horizons. Whether you're a seasoned soap artisan or just beginning your soapmaking adventure, each new recipe you create is an invitation to explore, experiment, and push the boundaries of what you know.

One of the most exciting aspects of soapmaking is the nearly limitless combination of ingredients you can incorporate. The interplay between different oils, butters, essential oils, and botanicals allows you to craft soaps tailored to specific needs and preferences.

While it's essential to grasp the basics first, the real magic happens when you mix, match, and innovate. Try experimenting with different superfatting levels to see how the excess oils affect moisturizing properties and soap texture. Don't be afraid to think outside the box and test unconventional ingredients—sometimes the most unexpected combinations yield the most delightful results.

As you delve deeper into the world of soapmaking, you'll find that keeping a detailed journal of your experiments is invaluable. Documenting your recipes, observations, and outcomes helps you understand how different variables impact the final product. Did adding a particular clay enhance the soap's lather? How did changing the water-to-lye ratio affect the soap's hardness? With meticulous notes, you can replicate successes and learn from any missteps, consistently improving your creations.

Aside from just mixing ingredients, exploring different techniques can elevate your soapmaking skills to new heights. Techniques like in-the-pot swirling, creating intricate layers, or embedding objects within the soap offer a playground of possibilities. Each method you master not only adds to your skillset but also makes your soaps more attractive and memorable whether for personal use or for sale.

Engaging with the broader soapmaking community can also be incredibly beneficial. Online forums, social media groups, and local workshops provide a wealth of knowledge and support from fellow enthusiasts. Sharing tips, seeking advice, and comparing notes can open new vistas for your soapmaking practice. Moreover, you can participate in challenges and collaborations that push you to experiment beyond your comfort zone, exposing you to fresh ideas and techniques.

An often overlooked but vital aspect of ongoing learning is seeking feedback. Constructive criticism from friends, family, and customers can provide valuable insights into both your strengths and areas for improvement. Are your scents too subtle? Are your soaps moisturizing enough? Listening to feedback not only helps you improve your formulations but also fosters a deeper connection with your audience, ensuring your soaps meet their needs and expectations.

Every soapmaker will eventually encounter batches that don't turn out as planned, and these moments are golden opportunities for learning. Did your soap seize unexpectedly, or did you end up with undesired colors? Troubleshooting such issues not only hones problem-solving skills but also deepens your understanding of the soapmaking process. Moreover, these experiences teach resilience and adaptability, which are crucial as you expand your soapmaking repertoire.

In addition to practical experience, continuous education through books, online courses, and workshops is essential. New research and emerging trends in soapmaking offer fresh perspectives and techniques. For example, the increasing availability of eco-friendly ingredients or advanced natural preservatives can significantly alter and improve your approach to soapmaking. Staying informed about these developments ensures your products remain both innovative and high-quality.

Moreover, don't underestimate the power of cross-disciplinary learning. Techniques and principles from other crafts, such as candle making, herbalism, or even culinary arts, can provide unique insights and inspiration. Understanding the properties of herbs and essential oils from an aromatherapeutic perspective, or learning about color theory from art, can add depth and dimension to your soapmaking practice.

Certainly, experimenting with different seasonal and themed soaps can be both fun and lucrative. Crafting holiday-specific batches or soaps designed for particular times of the year can attract a wider audience and imbue your soapmaking journey with a sense of rhythm and excitement. Imagine the joy of creating a pumpkin spice soap for autumn or a refreshing mint-scented bar for summer, each batch celebrating the essence of the season.

Developing a signature soap can also be a fulfilling venture, a flagship product that represents your unique style and expertise. Achieving this often involves extensive experimentation as you perfect every detail, from scent blend to texture. Your signature soap can become a hallmark of your brand, something that sets you apart in the crowded field of soapmakers.

Experimentation isn't just about the soap itself; it extends to your processes and operations. Playing with curing times, testing different mold styles and materials, or innovating your labeling and packaging can enhance both the product and the consumer's experience. Striving for sustainability within your soapmaking ensures your practices are in harmony with the eco-friendly ethos many soapmakers cherish.

Finally, continually remind yourself of why you started on this path. Whether it's the joy of creating, the pursuit of a cleaner lifestyle, or a desire to offer wholesome products to others, reconnecting with your purpose fuels your passion and curiosity. Each experiment, successful or otherwise, is a step forward on your soapmaking journey, an opportunity to learn, grow, and innovate.

Online Review Request for This Book

We'd love to hear about your soapmaking journey inspired by this book; please consider leaving an online review to share your thoughts and help others discover the joy of creating natural soaps with herbs and essential oils.

Conclusion

As we reach the conclusion of our journey into the world of natural soapmaking, it's heartening to reflect on the breadth and depth of the art we've explored together. From the humble beginnings of understanding the basics, to delving into advanced techniques and scaling up for business, this book has aimed to equip you with the knowledge and inspiration needed to create your own beautiful, natural soaps.

Soapmaking is more than just a craft; it's a journey towards sustainability, self-sufficiency, and creative expression. The process itself is transformative, converting simple ingredients into a product that cleanses, heals, and nurtures the skin. By choosing to craft your own soaps, you're not just making a product; you're embracing a lifestyle that values quality, natural ingredients, and eco-friendly practices.

Think back to where we started: understanding the history and evolution of soap. From ancient practices to modern advancements, soapmaking has always been a blend of science and art. Each bar of soap you create is a testament to that enduring legacy. You're now part of a tradition that spans millennia, one that has always adapted and thrived.

The practical chapters, replete with detailed instructions and safety guidelines, should now feel like a second nature. Whether it's the meticulous handling of lye or the precise calculations for perfect lye and oil ratios, these foundational skills ensure your soapmaking endeavors are not only successful but also safe. Your workspace, once perhaps daunting, is now a haven of creativity and productivity.

Yet, soapmaking also thrives on flexibility and innovation. Perhaps you've already begun experimenting with your own recipes, tweaking oil blends for the perfect lather, or infusing herbs and botanicals for that signature touch. The chapters on essential oils, natural colorants, and herbal additives are just the beginning of endless possibilities. The beauty of soapmaking lies in its adaptability—there's always room to explore new ideas and personalize your craft.

Your creativity isn't confined to just the ingredients. Designing intricate patterns, experimenting with textures, and creating themed seasonal soaps are expressions of your artistic vision. The skills you've acquired—from basic melt and pour techniques to advanced swirling and hot process methods—allow for endless customization. Each bar becomes a unique reflection of your artistry.

It's important to remember that soapmaking is a continuous learning process. Challenges like acceleration, ricing, and soda ash may still occur, but with experience and knowledge, you'll tackle these issues confidently. Embracing these challenges as opportunities for learning and growth will only enhance your skills and deepen your understanding of the craft.

For those looking to take their passion to the next level, perhaps even turning it into a business, the chapters on scaling up and selling your handmade soaps offer a roadmap. From sourcing sustainable materials to marketing your products effectively, these insights can transform a hobby into a viable enterprise. The emphasis on quality control and consistency ensures that your handcrafted soaps can stand out in any market.

The future of soapmaking is bright, filled with trends and innovations that continue to push the boundaries of what is possible.

Ethical sourcing, environmental sustainability, and creative collaborations are shaping the industry. By staying informed and connected with the soapmaking community through forums, workshops, and events, you'll be at the forefront of these exciting developments.

Finally, as you continue on your soapmaking journey, remember that there's always more to learn. The appendix and glossary serve as ongoing resources, while the broader community offers endless opportunities for inspiration and support. Whether you're improving your formulas or developing new products, continuous experimentation and education are key to staying engaged and inspired.

In conclusion, the world of natural soapmaking is as enriching as it is vast. It's a journey that nourishes not just the body, but the mind and soul. By combining tradition with innovation, and art with science, you've adopted a craft that is timeless yet ever-evolving. Your commitment to natural ingredients and sustainable practices contributes to a better future for both your customers and the planet.

Thank you for embarking on this journey and for your dedication to creating natural, handcrafted soaps. May your soapmaking endeavors bring joy, fulfillment, and a sense of accomplishment as you continue to explore and expand your skills.

The end is just the beginning. So, keep creating, keep experimenting, and most importantly, keep enjoying every step of the soapmaking process.

Appendix A: Resource Directory

In this Resource Directory, you'll find a comprehensive list of suppliers, organizations, and online communities that can provide you with the tools, ingredients, and knowledge necessary to elevate your soapmaking journey. Whether you're a seasoned soapmaker or just starting, these resources will help you find what you need.

Soapmaking Supplies and Ingredients

- **Bramble Berry** – Offers a wide range of soapmaking supplies, including oils, butters, molds, and fragrances. They also provide tutorials and recipes.
- **Wholesale Supplies Plus** – A one-stop shop for all your soapmaking needs, from raw materials to packaging supplies.
- **Soapgoods** – Specializes in natural and organic oils, butters, and essential oils perfect for your handmade soaps.
- **Nurture Soap** – Known for their vibrant colorants, molds, and other high-quality soapmaking supplies.
- **Bulk Apothecary** – Offers affordable soapmaking materials, including essential oils, base oils, and lye.

Essential Oils and Natural Additives

- **Mountain Rose Herbs** – A trusted source for organic herbs, essential oils, and natural additives.

- **New Directions Aromatics** – Provides a vast selection of essential oils and carrier oils at competitive prices.
- **Eden Botanicals** – High-quality essential oils and absolutes, perfect for aromatherapy and soapmaking.
- **Starwest Botanicals** – A reliable supplier of organic herbs, essential oils, and natural colorants.

Packaging and Presentation

- **Papermart** – Wide variety of packaging options, including boxes, wraps, and ribbons to beautifully present your handmade soaps.
- **SKS Bottle & Packaging** – Offers an extensive range of containers, jars, and labels for all your packaging needs.
- **Uline** – Known for their reliable shipping supplies and packaging materials.

Soapmaking Communities and Forums

- **Soapmaking Forum** – An active online community where soapmakers share tips, techniques, and advice.
- **Modern Soapmaking** – A blog and resource site with articles, tutorials, and a supportive community for soapmakers of all levels.
- **Facebook Groups** – Numerous groups such as "Soapmaking 101" and "Soapmaking for Beginners" where members can ask questions and share experiences.

Workshops and Certifications

- **Handcrafted Soap & Cosmetic Guild (HSCG)** – Offers certification programs, workshops, and an annual conference for soapmakers.
- **Soapmaking Studio** – Provides both online and in-person classes covering various soapmaking techniques and business aspects.

Books and Publications

- The Soapmaker's Companion by Susan Miller Cavitch – **A comprehensive guide for home soapmaking.**
- **Soap Crafting by Anne-Marie Faiola** – A book full of beautiful soap recipes and techniques from the founder of Bramble Berry.
- **Pure Soapmaking by Anne-Marie Faiola** – Features a variety of natural soap recipes using herbs and essential oils.

Online Learning and Tutorials

- **Soap Queen TV** – Video tutorials hosted by Anne-Marie Faiola, covering a wide range of soapmaking techniques and projects.
- **Lovin Soap Studio** – A blog with tutorials, recipes, and troubleshooting tips for both beginners and advanced soapmakers.

With these resources at your fingertips, you're well-equipped to embark on or continue your soapmaking adventure. Each source offers unique products, tips, and community support to help you create beautiful, natural soaps. Enjoy the exploration and happy soapmaking!

Glossary of Soapmaking Terms

Understanding the terminology used in soapmaking is key to mastering the craft. Here's a comprehensive list of soapmaking terms that you'll come across as you delve into this fascinating world:

A

- **Additive:** Any ingredient added to soap to enhance its properties, color, texture, or fragrance.
- **Alkali:** A substance with a high pH, such as lye (sodium hydroxide) or potassium hydroxide, that is essential in the soapmaking process for saponification.

B

- **Batch:** A single preparation of soap, typically referring to one mix of ingredients used to create multiple bars at once.
- **Base Oils:** The primary oils used in soapmaking, such as olive oil, coconut oil, and palm oil, which form the soap's foundation.
- **Bastille Soap:** A variant of Castile soap, typically made with at least 70% olive oil, but includes other oils as well.

C

- **Cure:** The period of time, usually 4-6 weeks, during which soap is allowed to rest and dry in order to complete the saponification process and become milder and harder.

- **Cylinder Mold:** A round mold used to create cylindrical soap bars.

E

- **Essential Oil:** A concentrated hydrophobic liquid containing volatile aroma compounds from plants, used to scent natural soaps.
- **Exfoliant:** An ingredient, such as seeds, salts, or powders, added to soap to provide scrubbing and exfoliating properties.

F

- **Fragrance Oil:** A man-made blend of synthetic or natural aromatic ingredients used to scent soap.

G

- **Gel Phase:** A part of the saponification process where the soap heats up and takes on a translucent, gel-like appearance.
- **Glycerin:** A natural by-product of saponification, glycerin is a humectant that attracts moisture to the skin.

H

- **Hot Process:** A soapmaking method where the soap mixture is heat-cooked to speed up saponification, resulting in a shorter curing time.

L

- **Layering:** The technique of pouring different layers of soap on top of each other, creating distinct stripes or patterns.

- **Lye:** A strongly alkaline solution (sodium hydroxide for bar soap, potassium hydroxide for liquid soap) that is essential for saponification.

M

- **Melt and Pour:** A pre-made glycerin soap base that can be melted, customized with additives and molded, bypassing the full saponification process.

O

- **Overheating:** When soap gets too hot during the curing process, potentially causing unwanted texture changes or cracks.

P

- **pH:** A measure of soap's acidity or alkalinity. Properly made soap typically has a pH of 9-10.
- **Potassium Hydroxide:** A type of lye used for making liquid soap.

S

- **Saponification:** The chemical reaction between oils (or fats) and lye to form soap and glycerin.
- **Superfatting:** The process of adding extra oil to the soap mixture, creating a more moisturizing final product.

T

- **Trace:** The point in the soapmaking process when the mixture thickens enough to leave a trace pattern on the surface.

W

- **Water Discount:** Reducing the amount of water in a soap recipe, which can speed up the curing process and produce a harder bar of soap.

This glossary will help you understand and navigate the terminology involved in soapmaking. As you continue your journey into creating natural soaps, refer back to these definitions whenever you need clarity on specific terms.

www.ingramcontent.com/pod-product-compliance
Lightning Source LLC
Chambersburg PA
CBHW031149020426
42333CB00013B/579